D0462210

CHIA
VITALITY

CHIA
VITALITY

• •

30 Days to Better Health, Greater Vibrancy,
and a More Meaningful and Purposeful Life

• •

JANIE HOFFMAN

HARMONY

BOOKS • NEW YORK

Published in the United States by Harmony Books, an imprint of the
Crown Publishing Group, a division of Random House LLC, New York,
a Penguin Random House Company. www.crownpublishing.com

Harmony Books is a registered trademark, and the Circle colophon is
a trademark of Random House LLC.

Library of Congress Cataloging-in-Publication Data
Hoffman, Janie.
  Chia vitality : 30 days to better health, greater vibrancy, and a more
meaningful and purposeful life / by Janie Hoffman.
     pages cm
1. Hatha yoga. 2. Vitality. I. Title.
  RA781.7.H64 2014
  613.7'046—dc23   2014000741

ISBN 978-0-8041-3978-6
eBook ISBN 978-0-8041-3979-3

Printed in the United States of America

Book design by Lauren Dong
Illustrations by Nicole Kaufman
Cover design by Jess Morphew
Cover photography: Gainey/Alamy

10 9 8 7 6 5 4 3 2 1

First Edition

Note to Reader

• • • • • •

This book is intended to provide helpful and inspirational information with the understanding that the author and publisher are not rendering medical, nutritional, or physical fitness services. Before starting on this (or any other) meal plan and exercise program, check with your physician to make sure that they will be right for you.

To Lance, my beautiful friend and delightful husband

Contents

......

CONTENTS

Introduction

· · · · · ·

LET CHIA CHANGE YOUR LIFE

vi·tal·i·t·y *noun—plural* **vi·tal·i·ties**
1. exuberant physical strength and mental vigor
2. capacity for the continuation of a meaningful and purposeful existence
3. power to live and grow
4. vital force

s there anyone who doesn't hunger for every single thing on that list? *Physical strength, mental vigor, a meaningful and purposeful existence, the power to live and grow, vital force* . . . Wow! That's a roster of just about everything sorely missing in most of our busy modern lives. Yet vitality and all that defines it isn't as elusive as it might seem. Even if you feel lacking in vitality right now, believe me, there's a vibrant, joyous person living inside you! You just need the right tools to bring it out—and chia is here to help.

When some people think about vitality, they think about having the energy to do more, and that's certainly a part of it. But when I think about vitality, I think about how it doesn't allow you to just *do* more—it allows you to *be* more. People with vitality are enthusiastic, passionate, and authentic. They're resilient in the face of life's ups and downs and filled with gratitude for the things, both big and small, that enrich their lives. Perhaps most notably, people with vitality are aligned with their soul's purpose. They've discovered what really matters to them and are living life accordingly. No wonder they feel so alive!

But can I get all that from a seed smaller than a freckle? You'd be right to be skeptical; when I first heard about the magic of chia, I was, too. It wasn't long, though, before I realized how well chia delivers on its promise—it's so much more than a nutrient-dense superfood. Seed by seed, this little powerhouse leads you down the path to vitality, giving you the energy and strength to lead a more beautiful and more dynamic life. Some foods simply feed the body, but chia also feeds the soul.

When you look at all that's packed into a single tablespoon of chia seeds, it's not hard to understand why there's a chia renaissance going on. Omega-3s! Fiber! Protein! Calcium! Iron! Antioxidants! And that's just a partial list. Gram for gram, there really isn't anything like chia: 70 percent more protein than soybeans, 25 percent more fiber than flaxseed, 600 percent more calcium than milk, and 30 percent more antioxidants than blueberries. Chia's omega-3 content alone— the highest of any vegetarian source—provides reason to celebrate. These essential fatty acids are known to protect the heart, help pre- vent cancer, reduce inflammation, diminish the symptoms of autoim- mune disorders, and possibly even guard against Alzheimer's disease and depression. And you get all that for a mere 60 to 68 calories per tablespoon (calories vary depending on who's doing the calculations,

SEEDS OF WISDOM

There is a vitality, a life force, an energy, a quickening, that is translated through you into action, and because there is only one of you in all time, this expression is unique.

—MARTHA GRAHAM, *modern dancer and choreographer*

but this is the general range). It's as if nature decided to develop its own wellness supplement—all the nutrients known to help fight disease and boost vigor conveniently packed into a small package, there for the taking.

When I talk about Mamma Chia, the chia-based food and beverage company I founded in 2009 and still run today, people sometimes ask if we use the same seeds that give Chia Pets their fluffy green hair, and they always smile when they learn that there is indeed a connection. Thanks to the Chia Pet folks, most people already have a good feeling about chia, and they know how to pronounce it! (Chia has thus escaped the fate of the poor acai [*ah-sigh-ee*] berry, which most people can never quite wrap their tongues around.) Until recently, though, most people had never used, let alone heard about using, chia as a food. But chia as a source of nutrition isn't so much a discovery as a *re*discovery. Hundreds of years before we had laboratory analyses to provide us with chia's nutritional stats, the Aztecs had detected its unrivaled restorative powers. They used chia for sustenance as well as for medicine and endurance. Aztec warriors would toss back a few spoonfuls of chia every few hours to give them the energy for battle and other demanding physical tasks. Even now, many runners are enamored of chia. The Tarahumara Indians, a native people of Mexico known for their long-distance running (they'll run for days, covering as much as two hundred miles), still use the seeds to power their marathon feats of athleticism.

Chia's invigorating health benefits make it the perfect catalyst for change. If you feel as if you're pedaling as fast as you can only to have the life you want elude you, this wellspring of vitality can help. It may seem like a stretch—how can a mere seed put you on the road to a more spirited and exuberant life?—but trust me, chia's like a shot in the arm. It wakes you up, giving you the mental clarity and physical energy you need to pursue your soul's purpose: a life with meaning, connection, and authenticity. That's the very definition of vitality!

At least that's my definition of vitality. These days, society seems to suggest that vitality is the ability to juggle a million things at once without flagging, to be endlessly productive, to get it all in—the clean diet, the five workouts a week, the organic garden in the backyard—and to just go, go, go, as abuzz as a hummingbird. I'd like to suggest that that's a by-product of too much coffee, not a definition of vitality. I believe it is time to drop the notion that it's easy to live a perfectly balanced life. I'm all for striving for balance, but striving for perfection has a way of undercutting the accomplishments we do achieve. In the pursuit of perfection, there's little room for being kind or forgiving of oneself, both essential to creating a vibrant, fulfilling life.

Chia Vitality is designed to set you free from the pressure to do it all. My goal is to get you to rethink what it means to be vital and alive—while also giving you the practical tools to achieve real vitality. To me, real vitality is the ability to feel centered and positive even when life is decidedly *unbalanced*. Real vitality is based on an acknowledgment that life has its ebbs and flows and that both can have equal value. It's the down moments in life that help prepare us for the ups, the calm that prepares us for the storm. In terms of real vitality, you can't have one without the other.

If you need to shake off fatigue, stress, overwork, and feelings of depletion—or if you simply want to hit the reset button on your lifestyle, this book is for you. But it's also meant to liberate you from unrealistic expectations. If you're tired of feeling guilty for missing a workout, anxious about straying from a "superclean" diet, remorseful about missing recycling day, ashamed about not being a do-it-all employee or parent, I hope you'll be heartened by this down-to-earth strategy for living.

In this 30-day plan, I'll introduce you to the wonders of chia while also showing you how it figures into an integrated, holistic plan for boosting vitality. Chia is not a magic bullet—no food is—but a chia-based diet can give you a fresh start and put you on the path to rejuvenation. I'll show you how you can combine chia with other, complementary strategies for nourishing body, mind, and soul, but first . . . a little backstory.

SEEDS OF WISDOM

. . . .

Vitality shows in not only the ability to persist but the ability to start over.

—F. SCOTT FITZGERALD, *author*

INSPIRATION!

I know what it feels like to be bursting with vitality. I also know what it feels like to be drained of every drop of vitality I've ever had. When I was in my early twenties, I began experiencing disturbing symptoms. I was feeling extreme fatigue and having difficulty dressing myself. There were times my muscles were so weak, I couldn't even get up from a chair. I had a bizarre rash on my face, chest, hands, and feet that wouldn't go away. I remember once going into a department store and being turned away by the salesperson at the cosmetics counter as soon as she caught sight of my rash. There was no way she was going to help me try on any makeup. I was a young woman not long out of college, newly married, a manager at a consumer products company—with an unsightly outbreak on my skin and barely enough energy to leave the house.

For a long time, my doctors couldn't even figure out what was wrong with me. The medical mystery was so confounding that I subjected myself to something called grand rounds, which involves checking in to the hospital and allowing over a hundred physicians, one or two at a time, to come into your room and offer their opinions. After their views—plus all kinds of muscle biopsies, skin biopsies, and blood tests—were tallied, I was finally diagnosed with a tongue twister of a condition called dermatomyositis. It's an uncommon autoimmune disorder that typically doesn't occur in adults until after age forty. There supposedly is no cure, but the disease can be put into remission. On my doctors' recommendation, I began taking a chemotherapy drug called methotrexate and the steroid prednisone, hoping that they could turn back the tide of total body depletion.

For the better part of two years I gave the drugs a fair shot. But I didn't respond positively to either. I had all the severe side effects—bloating and hair loss among them—and hardly any of the benefits. Worse, over the ensuing ten years I also acquired what's known as overlap syndrome. I kept coming down with one autoimmune disorder after another. After dermatomyositis came chronic fatigue, then lupus, then scleroderma, a scary hardening and contraction of the skin and connective tissue. When I got that last diagnosis, I had little to no movement of my scalp as well as significant hair loss.

Many doctors told me that there was just no getting completely well. "It's the name of the game with autoimmune disorders," they said. I still remember one doctor telling my husband and me that I was going to lose my hair and that there was nothing to be done about it. There were a lot of dispiriting conversations like that. I wasn't in denial, but I knew that there had to be something better that I could do. So, over the years, with traditional Western medicine unable to offer me much relief, I started looking elsewhere for help.

And if I couldn't have physical health, I decided I was going to attain greater spiritual health. My soul—that was the muscle I was going to develop! I began to study meditation and yoga in earnest, and I spent time volunteering for an AIDS organization, shuttling people in the last stages of the disease to and from their doctors' appointments.

During this time, I would go into remission for several months, only to experience devastating relapses or severe flare-ups. Have you ever worked out really hard—maybe you did more lunges or push-ups than ever before or ran five extra miles—and the next day your muscles protested with every move you made? That's what my auto-immune disorder symptoms felt like. I couldn't have felt worse if I'd been hit by a bus.

I also looked for other things I could do to try to heal myself: I adopted a strict vegan and macrobiotic diet for a year, but it didn't alleviate my symptoms any better than the drugs. I gave that up but continued to eat as healthfully as I could, consuming only organic foods whenever possible. Eating organically definitely helped more than anything else I had tried, and by 2009, I was having a pretty good run. I was even able to exercise on a regular basis.

One fateful day, I was working out with my friend Wendy when she mentioned chia. She excitedly reeled off a list of chia's benefits for me—omega-3s! fiber! protein! calcium! iron! antioxidants! (You'll see—these seeds inspire enthusiasm.) The list was so long I could scarcely believe it was true—or that I hadn't heard of chia sooner. I went home and started researching chia immediately. *Amazing!* I thought to myself as I paged through nutrient data and firsthand accounts of chia devotees. Even so, I had no idea that I would be in the chia business less than six months later—or that even before I launched Mamma Chia, my autoimmune disorders would be in total and complete remission.

My first supply of chia seeds was a small bag I ordered online. As soon as it came, I consumed about three tablespoons of the seeds, sprinkling them on my food throughout the day. As I said earlier, I'm not someone who believes in magic bullets. But after twenty years of listening closely to my body and trying to heal it in so many different ways, I know what works and what doesn't. *And there was no doubt about it.* The very first day I tried chia, I felt an increase in my vitality, energy, and strength. I began putting them in everything—and I've been doing so ever since. Within three months of making chia a daily part of my diet, I was totally free of any symptoms, and I haven't experienced one single flare-up since. I don't even test positive for autoimmune disorders anymore.

One of the things that made me so interested in chia in the first place was the link that studies found between higher omega-3 intakes and decreased symptoms of autoimmune diseases. Now my own personal experience was telling me that it was true. My home quickly became a chia laboratory. As my husband will attest, there wasn't a thing that came out of our kitchen that didn't have chia in it. Foods that were raw, foods that were cooked—all of them had chia seeds. Sometimes my husband would protest a little. "In ketchup? Really? Come on!"

I started carrying little snack bags of chia seeds everywhere so I could give them to people. And, although it never occurred to me at the time that it would turn into a commercial enterprise, I began making chia fruit drinks at home, pouring them into carafes and bringing them to yoga classes and dinner parties. By late summer 2009—just six months after I'd swapped flaxseeds for chia—I founded Mamma Chia. Off to a brilliant start!

Or so I thought. I quickly discovered that my kitchen recipes didn't translate well in production. We had one disastrous test run after another and were told over and over again that it couldn't be done. But I was determined to spread my love of chia through my unique chia beverages. Eventually, we made it work. It was an incredibly joyous day when Mamma Chia landed on Whole Foods' shelves in October 2010. Mamma Chia was the first chia-based beverage on the market; in fact, it created a whole new category of beverages and (thankfully) was met with great success.

Now I want to bring the magic of chia to you as part of a comprehensive program that will increase effervescence in all areas of your life. If there was one thing I learned during those years I spent struggling with autoimmune disorders, it's that you can't take your body for granted. It's a gift to have physical exuberance, and well worth your while to work on gaining and maintaining it. But we are not just our physical bodies. If during those years of being unable to gracefully pull on a shirt or agilely get up from a chair I believed physical energy was the be-all and end-all, I would have been a lost soul. Cultivating my inner life gave me an emotional, mental, and spiritual energy that allowed me to feel vital regardless of my level of physical vigor.

WHAT LIES IN STORE

Nothing can change the way you feel like changing the way you eat. If you switch from a diet of junk and fast food to a diet rich in barely processed whole foods, you'll feel the difference immediately. In the same way, working chia into your diet will make your body stand up and take notice. And that will happen no matter where you're coming from—whether you already eat mainly nutritious foods or you could stand to clean up your act.

Of all the many reasons I've become chia's number one fan, the most important is this: chia is a *food*. That, I know, is stating the obvious, but think about it. Chia is a beautiful, natural, unadulterated product of the earth that offers us the gift of good health. It's not a supplement made by extracting nutrients from their source; it's the source itself. I'm not a technophobe—I believe in progress, really I do!—but some things in life should be simple, and how we nourish our bodies is one of them.

I've designed a 30-day meal plan to help introduce you to the wonders of chia. This plan is built on a platform of flavorful whole foods that bring health benefits of their own to the table. It's easy to follow and is flexible. Breakfasts can be swapped with other breakfasts, snacks switched with other snacks, and lunches or dinners exchanged with other lunches or dinners to suit your tastes. You can also control the portion sizes based on your own particular needs. And if you need a jump start, there's an optional three-day cleanse that can help you make the transition to chia-based eating.

The main objective isn't to stress you out with strict dietary rules or difficult recipes, but rather to simply help you increase your intake of omega-3s, fiber, protein, antioxidants, and all the other vitality-boosting nutrients that chia has to offer. My goal is to familiarize you with all the ways chia can be incorporated into your life and to help you make chia eating a habit.

One of the reasons I'm so crazy about chia is that it offers so much but asks so little of you. You don't have to go to the ends of the earth to buy it. You don't have to consume it at particular times of day or knock yourself out preparing it in special ways. There's no grinding or fermenting. You don't even have to cook chia, though of course it makes a great addition to all kinds of dishes, as you'll see in the *Chia Vitality* recipes in chapter 9.

The *Chia Vitality* eating plan isn't a weight loss diet per se, but it has elements that may help you slim down if you want to. When chia is hydrated, it forms a gel-like coating that can help you feel fuller and eat fewer calories. The *Chia Vitality* plan is also chock-full of protein and fiber, both of which are known to help with weight loss.

I want to help you learn to experiment with chia. Besides filling you in on chia's history and how it fits into the picture that health experts and researchers have painted of omega-3s, this book has numerous tips and tricks for using chia to its fullest (you might, for instance, be surprised to learn that you can use chia to substitute for eggs in baking). My own kitchen looks like a scientist's lair. I've always got jars of hydrated chia in my refrigerator that can be used as a base for all kinds of things—Caesar salad dressing, puddings, stir-fry flavorings, and both fruit and green vegetable smoothies. The possibilities are endless.

As you are making the shift to a chia-based diet, you can also begin to add in the other vitality-enhancing elements of this program. Not surprisingly, the first one is exercise. There's no doubt that moving your body is a critical piece of staying fit and healthy. But its contribution to increasing vitality is often undervalued. The *Chia Vitality* approach to exercise allows you to capitalize on the endurance-boosting benefits of chia (talk about a double whammy—chia gives you energy so you can get even more of it through exercise) by helping you find the workouts that suit you best. If you think of exercise as something that tires you out rather than revs you up, you are probably working out in a way that's not right for your body.

As a longtime practitioner of yoga, I have found it to be both soothing and invigorating—it gets at vitality from both sides and helps align the body with the soul. And, contrary to what's often assumed, yoga is something just about everyone can do. I'll introduce you to the *Chia Vitality* yoga practice, a short, simple routine for building flexibility and strength that also has quite a bit else to offer. The *Chia Vitality* yoga practice can help you work in a quick session of activity every day—one you can do anywhere, anytime—but perhaps even more important, it also gives you an opportunity to expand your consciousness and gain a deeper awareness and understanding of who you truly are.

The third element of this program is mindful meditation. If you're someone who balks at the idea of sitting alone in a room cross-legged while chanting for forty-five minutes, don't worry: that's not the kind of meditation I'm talking about. Mindfulness, which can be practiced while walking, eating, or even washing the dishes, is intended to help you pay attention to the present moment and be observant—of your life, your thoughts, the world around you—without judgment. Judgment saps vitality; it's being more accepting of yourself and others that helps give you the buoyancy to bounce joyfully through life. There is no religion or dogma attached to mindfulness, but it *is* spiritual. And while it may seem to have nothing to do with upping your intake of omega-3s and antioxidants, it is a logical counterpart to a chia-based diet. By following the *Chia Vitality* plan, you'll be making an effort to eat more consciously. Mindful meditation will help you live more consciously, too.

Something I consider part of the practice of mindfulness is gratitude. Gratitude—actively acknowledging the things, big and small, that enrich your life—not only leads to greater satisfaction, it also helps you let go of trying to control everything. We all know that life has challenges; what the practice of gratitude does is enable you to trust that those challenges are moving you toward your highest and best self. With a practice of gratitude, life becomes more wondrous and exciting. And gratitude helps you stay steady when the waves of life inevitably rock your boat.

It's not a far leap from mindfulness to thinking about reaching out to others in the world around you. I've made expanding your world a part of this 30-day plan because, while vitality comes from within, being part of a wider community can give you energy and purpose. One of the ways I coped with my autoimmune disorders in those early days was by seeing what I could do to help better the world around me. Even just being part of a group of like-minded yoga practitioners helped make me feel more full of life. And we know that being part of a community has health benefits. People who reach out live longer and have lower rates of depression and heart disease. I'll have some suggestions on how you can increase your sense of feeling part of a greater whole.

The tagline placed on all Mamma Chia products is "Seed Your Soul," and it seems to me that it's also a suitable description for *Chia Vitality*. In the next 30 days you'll be doing more than feeding your body with the bountiful nutrients in chia: You'll be seeding your soul by going inward and moving outward. You'll think less about finding perfect balance and more about being perfectly happy in your own skin. And you'll take steps to ensure that you not only feel strong and energetic right now, but well into the future. Chia is your gateway to lifelong vitality!

1

· · · · · · ·

SETTING THE COURSE
FOR VITALITY

When I first started Mamma Chia and began speaking in public, I was very reluctant to share the story of my struggles with autoimmune disorders. I wanted to focus just on the amazing properties of the chia seeds themselves. But, inevitably, people would ask me why I was so passionate about these little seeds, and slowly I became more comfortable telling my story. As a result, many of the people I spoke to opened up and shared tales of their health struggles or spoke about their strong desire for well-being. Sometimes, like me, they'd grappled with severe illness. Sometimes they just felt lackluster. Sometimes they were looking for the boost that would make them a better athlete or help them achieve more at work or school. Whatever their needs, I know that most of them were hoping I'd say that chia was a miracle food—the magic bullet they'd been searching for.

There *is* magic to chia—I'm certain of that, and you're about to learn all about what makes it so special. But as much as I hated to disappoint searchers looking for an easy solution, I had to tell them that there were many aspects to my recovery and my supercharged vitality. Yoga, meditation, an organic diet of whole foods, and service—all the things I will talk about in the pages of this book—also played a role in helping me go into remission and have the strength and energy to initiate and sustain a demanding business. In fact, I think I'm living proof that synergy—you might also call it an integrative or holistic approach—yields great results. Synergy gave birth to my present good health and the fulfilling work I do as CEO and founder of Mamma Chia.

Once you get to know me, you'll notice that I tend to see many things through a chia lens. Okay, so maybe once in a while I go overboard, but it often makes complete sense. For instance, I think of chia as a perfect metaphor for the synergistic approach to vitality that I just described. Chia gets its power to boost energy, stamina, physical strength, and resistance to disease not from just one nutrient—say, omega-3s or protein—but from the *combined potency* of the many nutrients packed into those tiny seeds. In the same way, you'll become truly vital through the integration of eating well, moving your body, awakening your soul, reaching out to the world, and letting gratitude and kindness guide you. The joie de vivre we're all aiming for can never be achieved by paying attention only to one aspect of your being. So if you're curious as to why this book goes beyond just familiarizing you with chia, there's your answer: to get you on the path to a more vibrant, meaningful, and purposeful existence, I want to introduce you to *all* the things I've found to be life changing and that complement a chia-based diet so well. That's what works best, so why not go for it all?!

I, of course, am not the only one who believes in a synergistic, holistic, and integrative approach to well-being. There is more and more evidence that addressing the body, mind, *and* spirit in a variety of different ways is optimal for almost all aspects of good health and vitality. It's no accident that the number of integrative medical programs around the country is increasing. And these are not far-flung, hole-in-the-wall outposts, but rather wellness programs at mainstream universities and medical centers. Stanford, the University of Maryland, Duke University, the University of California at San Francisco, and the University of California at San Diego are just some of the prominent schools that now also take an integrative approach to well-being. Think of the multifaceted 30-day plan you're about to embark on as joining the ranks of these progressive thinkers.

REDEFINING VITALITY

The word *vitality* is often used interchangeably with the word *energy*, but to me the two are not the same. Although energy is most certainly a *component* of vitality, having vitality involves more than just being able to ward off fatigue and approach life with mental and physical vigor. True vitality goes deeper—and wider.

When you picked up this book, you no doubt had an idea of what you hoped to achieve. So what's your definition of *vitality*? I'll tell you mine. I think of it as the ability to be your authentic self, to follow your passions, and to feel connected to the people and the world around you. Instead of living a passive existence, people who sparkle with vitality are deeply and purposefully engaged in life. They zero in on what matters to them, feel grateful for what they have, and celebrate the present moment. And when they hit a rocky patch in life, which is inevitable, people with vitality have the strength, resilience, and wherewithal to remember "This too shall pass." It even causes them to take a deeper dive into gratitude, opening more doors to vitality and joy.

If that inventory of qualities sounds daunting, keep in mind that vitality is not so much a list of accomplishments you must check off as an attitude and a way of life. Vitality is rooted in *mindfulness*, a term you'll see repeatedly in this book. There's mindful meditation, which I'll introduce you to in chapter 6, and there's mindfulness as it applies to our everyday lives. The two are related, but for now let's talk about everyday mindfulness.

Mindfulness is awareness—awareness of your body, your thoughts, your feelings, your environment, and the people around you. It's walking to the bus stop and, instead of just putting your head down and going full speed ahead, it's noticing that the trees' leaves are turning golden in the fall air. It's noticing that you feel a wave of anger rising when someone takes the parking space you've been waiting for and, instead of just seething, it's acknowledging the fact that you're feeling angry (try it—there's a difference between the two) and consciously letting it go. It's not just looking at but *seeing* the checker who's totaling up your groceries and the guy you pass on your way to work each day and giving them a little smile or a wave. When you are completely alert and accepting of all that is going on inside and around you, life is richer. Mindfulness also gives you the opportunity to catch things that need your attention—such as how you could have let losing a parking space ruin your day or how that little smile and wave brighten your morning.

To me, our awareness should be expansive and inclusive, encompassing mindfulness of the planet and all the people who inhabit it. I don't mean that you must mull over climate change and the human condition every moment of the day, but I find that being conscious of life beyond yourself and your immediate friends and family brings an energizing feeling of interconnectedness—an understanding on a deeper level that you are part of the world and the world is part of you.

Mindfulness also allows you to become attuned to yourself on a deeper level, making you more conscious of your actions, thoughts, and feelings. To some degree, we all operate on autopilot, without paying attention to what we're doing. We may also ignore signals we're getting from our bodies and even tamp down emotions rather than acknowledge that our inner lives need attending to. For instance, many people often exercise too much or too little, choose the wrong workouts, eat past fullness, and consume food that's unhealthful or even damaging, all without regard to how physically uncomfortable those things are making them feel. Sometimes it's also easy to disregard or discount hurt feelings or discontent until they become so

toxic you feel you're ready to explode—and sometimes do, jeopardiz-
ing or damaging your relationships or sending you into a downward
spiral of guilt and shame. By helping you continually to "check in,"
to listen to your body's intuitive wisdom, and to heighten your own
sense of yourself, mindfulness helps you avoid many of the things that
sap vitality. When you're fully awake and aware, it becomes easier to
make good choices and to live the healthy, dynamic life you are meant
to live.

There are two other elements of vitality I'd like to elaborate on.
One is discovering and living your "soul's purpose," a phrase you'll see
me use throughout this book. Each one of you has a soul's purpose.
Your soul—the reality of who you truly are, your deepest self apart
from any outside influences or pressures—has a unique purpose to
fulfill. When you are in alignment with your soul's purpose, you feel
it! You are in the zone. And you are able to face each moment with
more enthusiasm, joy, passion, openness, optimism, and authenticity.
Now that's pure vitality!

Most of us can't always live in perfect alignment with our soul's
purpose—I know I certainly haven't mastered that yet. But maybe
that's because we're too busy trying to be perfect. (Perfectionism, as
I'll elaborate on shortly, is the enemy of vitality!) You can, however,
learn to achieve greater alignment between your soul and your personality. And when you do, all kinds of miraculous things happen. You
become more mindful of the immense beauty in the world around
you, and it fills you with awe (alignment with your soul helps you to
be more mindful, and mindfulness helps you align with your soul's
purpose—it's a lovely little circle). You become more easygoing as well
as more kind and forgiving of yourself and others. Your capacity for
joy is heightened in a way that even the tiniest of pleasures can bring
great contentment. Who doesn't need more of that?!

Finally, I'd like to talk about gratitude, which I mentioned briefly
in the introduction to this book. Nothing can help you move through
life with more grace and ease than gratitude. When you feel thankful
for all things, big and small, it allows you to embrace your life as it

actually is, not how you wish it to be. Gratitude—and I'll talk more about how to practice it in chapter 6—takes a weight off your shoulders and renews your energy and spirit. And, as I found out when my health reached its lowest point, there is always *something* to be thankful for.

It's important not to confuse gratitude with complacency. You can be grateful for all that you have and everything that crosses your path and still have a drive to reach goals you set for yourself. In fact, I believe that practicing gratitude attracts things to you that help you reach your goals. (When I first discovered chia, I wrote in my gratitude journal, which I still keep to this day, "I'm grateful for the vitality I felt all day today—I know it's the chia." And see, Mamma Chia came my way!) Practicing and cultivating gratitude is different from the power of positive thinking. I don't really subscribe to the "think only positive thoughts and only positive things will happen to you" theory of life. Who doesn't know some wonderfully positive person who was hit by heartache or tragedy? Illness, sadness, and misfortune all occur whether we continually stay cheery or not. Gratitude doesn't keep bad things from happening, but it does help you stay strong, resilient, and endlessly vital.

SEEDS OF WISDOM

What is joy without sorrow? What is success without failure? What is a win without a loss? What is health without illness? You have to experience each if you are to appreciate the other. There is always going to be suffering. It's how you look at your suffering, how you deal with it, that will define you.

—MARK TWAIN, *author and humorist*

THE MYTH OF PERFECT BALANCE

Now that you have an idea of what my definition of vitality is, let's talk about what vitality *isn't*: namely, a life that's both perfect and perfectly balanced. We hear a lot about "balance" these days, which to me is just a euphemism for "doing it all." Eat right and exercise. Have a fulfilling job, but don't burn the midnight oil at the expense of your health, family, and friends. Recycle. Volunteer. Maybe even grow your own food. It all sounds wonderful, and it is—I'm for all of these things. But trying to live a life that's balanced often means that you're being pulled in a hundred different directions rather than giving necessary attention to any one area of your life. Two of the hallmarks of vitality are passion and commitment, but it's difficult to focus on what you're passionate about and committed to when your mental and physical energy is split among so many things. See what I mean about perfectionism being the enemy of vitality! The enormous effort of trying to keep so many balls in the air without letting one single ball drop can suck the life right out of you.

Given the undue pressure we're all under to take on responsibilities and rack up accomplishments, it's hard not to beat yourself up about, say, eating foods that aren't perfectly "clean," letting your gym membership go unused, or having the holidays at home instead of volunteering at a soup kitchen. Suddenly, not composting seems like a moral failure. And it's very easy to fall into the trap of trying to keep up with the Joneses or wanting (and trying) to look like someone else. We might blame these outsized expectations on society, or on our parents, or on the internal convictions we developed somewhere down the line—the origins don't really matter. Whatever the source, the feeling of not measuring up to our own or others' expectations can be disheartening. That's why, as part of pursuing a life with greater vitality, it's so important to get a clear sense of your own priorities. Rather than feeling as though you must do it all, pace yourself.

This is the moment to take a step back from the obligations and responsibilities that fill your life and ask yourself: What are my real priorities? What's most meaningful to me? What will enhance my life most? What is my soul's purpose? Try to identify the two or three things that really matter to you: those should be where your focus and energy go. Sure, other things will have to give, but not necessarily forever. Finish with one or a few things, then take on the next that brings you closer to your soul's purpose.

One thing I think we all know intuitively—but that often gets lost in the shuffle of trying to achieve perfect balance—is that life has natural ebbs and flows. There may be times when life is flowing so fast that you feel as if you're drinking from a fire hose! It's intense, but it can be wonderful, too. Ebbs can be just the opposite, a drip, drip, drip so meager you hardly feel you are getting any sustenance from what life is handing you. Sometimes life gives you lemons, and sometimes life gives you lemonade, and each has its value. Vitality springs from being able to roll with the times, taking all you can from each experience and being forgiving of yourself when you can't do all that you want or hope to. Return your focus to your priorities and forget about being perfect! I like what the nineteenth-century British social thinker and art critic John Ruskin said about those times we often perceive as too flawed to have merit: "To banish imperfection is to destroy expression, to check exertion, to paralyze vitality." Exactly!

Not long ago, I found myself living what might be considered a very imperfect life; it certainly was out of whack. It occurred during the period I was bringing Mamma Chia to fruition. I spent months, too many to count, working eighteen-plus hours a day. That left no room for balance, no room for practically anything else—just ask my husband, Lance, who had toast for dinner more times than I can count. I barely ever exercised, and meditation, long a staple in my life, had shrunk down to the bare minimum. But because I was following my passion, I also had never felt more alive! I think this is a good example of how placing your focus where it needs to be at any given

SEEDS OF WISDOM

What you focus on grows. If we only focus on what's not working, we're cheated of the joy, satisfaction, relaxation, and peace that comes with seeing the whole picture.

—ELIZABETH CROOK, *creator of Discover Your Yippee!*

time, even if it means your life is imbalanced and that other things you care about may need to take a temporary backseat, can lead to greater fulfillment, energy, and joy.

Sometimes you have to take a deep dive into one aspect of your life. It could be the job you have now; it could be caring for children or other members of your family; it could be training for a marathon; it could be a creative endeavor; it could be starting a new nonprofit or a business—it could be anything you're passionate about or know in your soul is the right thing to do. The point is, something will have to give, and that's okay. Think of all you will get from following your soul's purpose and know that you will come back closer to a place of "balance" when you can.

CREATING A FOUNDATION FOR VITALITY

Once Mamma Chia had found its footing, my husband and I were able to resume our evening dinners together (at least when I wasn't on the road traveling). I returned to many of the other important things in my life that had fallen by the wayside at the height of Mamma Chia mania, including practicing more yoga and meditating for longer periods of time again. What made regaining a life of greater equilibrium easier was the fact that I had a foundation of healthy practices to come back to. It also helped that Lance and I had built a solid partnership based on friendship and service, one offering an emotional and spiritual foundation to bolster us when our lives might become more difficult. Dedicating our life to service and anticipating that life has its regular ups and downs, we even wrote that foundation into our marriage contract. This excerpt from our contract says it all:

> *We have entered into a new dimension of our relationship, a relationship which when qualified by love and wisdom, offers not only an enhancement of that love, but also a greater field of service within the One Life. This service to which we are joined is the reflection of God into our daily life and affairs, the environment, and outward into humanity, thus helping to lift the soul of all who come within our influence.*
>
> *We declare our intention to give one another our deepest friendship and love, not only when our moments are high, but when they are low; not only when we remember clearly who we are, but when we forget; not only when we are acting with love, but when we are not.*

One of the goals of this book is to help you lay the bricks of a vitality foundation so it's easier to find your way back from times when leading a balanced life is impossible. It's a bit of a catch-22, I know: Here I am telling you that it's not always possible to achieve perfect balance, but I am inviting you to follow a perfectly balanced 30-day plan. It may sound a little crazy, but hear me out. What I'm asking is that you take the next 30 days to live with your own vitality as your priority. Maybe you won't eat a chia-based diet every day of your life; maybe your yoga or preferred mode of fitness will fall by the wayside from time to time; and maybe you won't always meditate or reach out to your community. It happens. But once you have experienced how buoyant and vibrant you feel when all those healthy components are in place, you'll know you can come back to them whenever you need them—and you will. Taking these 30 days to establish a foundation of vitality will stand you in good stead both now and later down the line. During those times when life spins out of control, you can take comfort—and judge yourself less harshly for not living as you know you "should"—because you have learned how to use the tools that will help you refocus and replenish your life.

Here's something I think can also add to the foundation you're building: a list of your core values. Most businesses have a mission statement and some (like Mamma Chia) have a list of core values, too. I think individuals can also benefit from creating a list of what they need in order to give meaning and purpose to their lives. The list can be very specific, or it can just outline some general tenets. Here, for instance, are seven that I think represent the heart and soul of vitality:

1. Cultivate physical, emotional, and spiritual well-being.
2. Be unabashedly passionate about what you love.
3. Build meaningful and delightful relationships.
4. Strive for excellence (not perfection).
5. Awaken to the world around you and the soul within you, and offer yourself in service.
6. Be all in when life flows; accept and learn from the ebbs.
7. Practice unconditional compassion and kindness to yourself and others.

See the exercise on page 12 to create your own list of core values.

SEEDS OF WISDOM

If you look for perfection, you'll never be content.

—LEO TOLSTOY, *Russian novelist*

PLANT YOUR SEEDS OF VITALITY

I believe that vitality comes from being true to yourself, and being true to yourself means giving priority to those things that mesh with your values and give your life purpose. So what are the things you value? What is it that gives your life purpose? Let's find out! Get out a sheet of paper and write down answers to the questions below. Then spend some time going over what you wrote. Winnow your answers down to seven or eight concepts, and use those to make your list of core values in the style of the one I offer on page 11.

1. What brings you joy?
2. What ignites your passion?
3. What do you love to do?
4. What makes you laugh out loud?
5. What are your natural gifts?
6. How would you want to share those gifts with the world?
7. What do you need to do to be more kind and compassionate to yourself and others?
8. Whom do you enjoy spending the most time with?
9. If money and time were not a concern, what would you do?
10. What character traits do you appreciate most about yourself?
11. What changes do you want to see in the world?
12. When do you feel the most alive?
13. Who are the people you admire, and what are their attributes?
14. What makes you feel the most fulfilled and renewed—physically, mentally, and spiritually?

Your answers to these questions should give you a snapshot of what's most important to you and what energizes and delights you. Make those things the focus of your core values list.

GOING FORWARD

The pathways to vitality you'll find in this book are essentially activities—eating well, moving your body, meditating, getting involved. But as much as they're about actively *doing* something, they're really about self-discovery and reframing the way you think. It goes back to one of the definitions of vitality I mentioned at the beginning of this book: *the capacity for the continuation of a meaningful and purposeful existence.* Throughout these next 30 days, use each element of the *Chia Vitality* plan to explore what it is that makes you feel the most effervescent and that ignites your soul's purpose. Set aside all the expectations—yours and others—and let your true self come to the surface. Listen to your body, listen to your soul. Replace negative talk with more compassion and acceptance. Love what is. That's how you'll discover what nourishes you physically and emotionally, resonates with your intellect, and is in alignment with the purpose of your soul. That, in short, is going to give you vitality to spare!

SEEDS OF WISDOM

Do stuff. Be clenched, curious. Not waiting for inspiration's shove or society's kiss on your forehead. Pay attention. It's all about paying attention. Attention is vitality. It connects you with others. It makes you eager. Stay eager.

—SUSAN SONTAG, *writer and activist*

2

. . . .

GOOD THINGS COME IN

SMALL PACKAGES

Everyone is looking for more mojo. Punishing schedules, long working hours, financial pressures, traffic, pollution, meals that don't truly nourish: the times we live in can sap your energy, not to mention your soul. So it's no surprise that when people hear about chia's vitality-enhancing powers, their ears perk up. And the word is spreading. *Bloomberg Businessweek* called chia the "stimulant of choice" on Wall Street, where hard-driving Gordon Gekko types are stirring chia into yogurt with their right hand while moving money across markets with their left. According to the *Wall Street Journal,* chia is also the National Football League's "top-secret seed." Don't you just love the image of 212-pound rusher Ray Rice scooping up the minuscule seeds in his big hands and sprinkling them on his food? Powerhouse meets powerhouse!

As someone who aspires to be the Johnny Appleseed of chia, spreading seeds of good health wherever I go, I am happy anytime I hear that chia is making inroads with one group or another. But make no mistake about it: chia is not a fad. It's not a fashionable food that will be here today, gone the way of oat bran tomorrow. Chia is the real deal! You just have to glance at its nutritional profile to know that these seeds are too powerful and too easy to integrate into your diet to ever fall by the wayside.

The story of chia—from the bygone halls of Montezuma to the contemporary halls of Lower Manhattan—is also a story about how our relationship with food has evolved. As it turns out, what ancient people knew intuitively and through nonscientific forms of trial and error has been confirmed by modern nutritional analysis. Wisdom was lost, but as the chia story shows (and fortunately for us), wisdom can be regained. Let's start at the beginning.

SEEDS OF KNOWLEDGE

WHAT'S IN CHIA'S NAME?

The Aztecs called chia *chian*, and somewhere along the way, the *n* was lopped off. (*Chia* in Nahuatl, the Aztec language, actually means "to wait.") "The other Nahuatl word for the seed was *chiyantli*, which connotes the idea of oil," says John F. Schwaller, a professor of history at the State University of New York, Potsdam, and an expert in the Aztecs' native language. When I was researching the origins of the word *chia*, I stumbled across another translation of the word. In Vietnamese, *chia* means "share." It's unrelated to the seed, but how perfect is that? Chia is something you definitely want to share with others.

CHIA'S VENERABLE PAST

Where have these seeds been all my life? Like finding the perfect love after years of so-so relationships, I wish that I'd met chia seeds sooner. *They're so great,* I thought after a few weeks of using them and marveling at their effects; *why haven't I heard of them before?* It's not as though chia is some hybrid plant that clever farmers cooked up in their fields in an effort to entice new customers. Nor is chia a genetically modified organism (GMO) that some big corporation concocted in its labs. In fact, people have been eating chia (*Salvia hispanica*), a member of the mint family (Lamiaceae), for eons—perhaps as early as 3500 BC, according to agriculture historians. But except in Latin America, where chia has long been part of the culinary vernacular, these mighty seeds have largely been overlooked.

It wasn't always so. Before the arrival of Columbus, chia was once a major commodity in Mesoamerica, the region that extends from central Mexico down through Belize, Guatemala, El Salvador, Honduras, Nicaragua, and northern Costa Rica. The seeds were likely a staple of several of the flourishing civilizations that lived in the area, but thanks to firsthand accounts and historical documents written primarily by the Spanish, we know quite a bit about how the Aztecs used chia. And were they crazy for the stuff! They ate it, of course—often combined with other grains to form a flour known as *chianpinolli,* which they'd then use to make tortillas and tamales. They used chia in beverages, too, adding *chianpinolli* to water (sometimes with chiles) to create a drink called *chiantole,* a precursor to *chia fresca* and *agua de chia,* the drinks sold by vendors on the streets of Mexico today.

To the Aztecs, though, chia was more than just a form of basic sustenance. They also saw it as what we might call a "functional food"— a food with therapeutic powers. University of Arizona researchers Ricardo Ayerza Jr. and Wayne Coates, who have made an exhaustive study of chia's history, report that Aztec warriors carried small bags of corn and chia flour the way modern soldiers might carry energy bars or Gatorade. They'd combine the chia with water and syrup to create a hydrating, stimulating pick-me-up. Returning from battle, weary soldiers would be revived with bowls of chia porridge before being sent out to face the enemy once again.

Chia was used as medicine, too. The seeds (and sometimes other parts of the plant) were used to treat gastrointestinal and respiratory ills, reduce fever, and soothe burns. The Chumash Indians, natives of Southern California, were known to use seeds to remove sand or other obstructions from the eyes. They'd lift the lid, place a few seeds underneath, and allow the gel to catch the offending particle (probably best not to try this at home!). When traveling on long journeys, another group of California natives, the Diegueño, would tuck a few chia seeds in their mouths and chew them periodically for energy—one tablespoon was said to bestow twenty-four hours' worth of get-up-and-go. The Aztecs turned chia oil into body paint and lacquer for preserving clay vessels. They considered the seeds a form of currency, requiring that the city-states they'd conquered pay them tributes—taxes, essentially—in the way of baskets of chia. Chia figured into religious ceremonies as well, as an offering to the gods.

Chia's religious significance may be one reason the crop nearly died out. When the Spanish conquered the Aztecs, they were appalled by the Aztecs' spiritual practices and had particular contempt for foods that figured into religious rites. They destroyed many of the natives' crops, then forced them to cultivate and tend European staples such as wheat and barley.

And yet chia did survive. While much of the Aztec civilization was wiped out by diseases brought by the Europeans, some who survived isolated themselves in parts of Southwestern Mexico and Guatemala and continued to keep many of their traditions alive, as did their descendants. One of those traditions was the cultivation and consumption of chia, although the keepers of the flame didn't use the seeds as expansively as their forebears. Instead, chia seeds have primarily been used in the drinks *chia fresca* and *aqua de chia,* though they are sometimes still integrated into food and sold as medicine, too.

One group of Indians, the Tarahumara, who live in the Copper Canyon of Northwest Mexico, also maintained the tradition of using chia for energy. Known for their epic runs—some lasting hundreds of miles—the Tarahumara fuel themselves with a chia brew known as *iskiate,* made by hydrating the seeds in a little water, then adding a touch of sugar and a squeeze of lime.

When I think about the Aztecs' story, I think about how clearly it illustrates what's been lost (or nearly lost) in modern agriculture. It seems as though with each succeeding generation, we've turned further away from the nutritionally rich plants that sustained our ancestors so well. With all the industrial farming that goes on today, many of the fruits, vegetables, and grains reaching our tables, bred for their

ability to withstand transport and look good stacked up in the produce aisle, offer very little in the way of healthy vitamins, minerals,
omega-3s, and phytochemicals. Once, when scientists compared wild
tomatoes to the supermarket variety, they found that the wild ones
had 40 more times the amount of lycopene, an important phytonutri-
ent. Some wild varieties of apples have been found to have as much
as 65 to 100 times the levels of phytonutrients as their commercial
counterparts. Chia represents a return to basics.

NUTRIENTS GALORE! CHIA'S
EXTRAORDINARY HEALTH PROFILE

What you eat is key to how exuberant you feel. Eat junky food and
you're going to be dragging around, moody and weak. Eat nutritious
food and you're going to feel strong, light, alert, and ready to take on
the world. It's as simple as that. Food, when it's right, works magic.

But as much as I'm over the moon about chia, I'm not telling you
to take two tablespoons and call me in the morning. While chia can
up your vitality quotient substantially, it can't necessarily do it all by
its itty-bitty self. Chia elevates your diet in the same way that, say, a
beautiful sofa takes a nice living room to the next level. The living
room was fine before, but now it's something really, really amazing. I've
talked about how chia works as part of an integrative lifestyle approach
to boosting vitality. Well, it also works as part of an integrative eating approach: add chia to a diet of varied, nutrient-rich, unprocessed,
and preferably organic foods, and you're filling your body with what it
needs to protect your health, boost your energy, and nourish your soul.

In 2013, researchers at the Laboratory of Food Biotechnology,
part of Mexico's Center for Research and Advanced Studies of the
National Polytechnic Institute (CINVESTAV), analyzed chia seeds.
The report of their results, published in the *Journal of Agricultural
and Food Chemistry*, called chia an important source of protein and
highlighted its high content of oil rich in omega-3s. The researchers

were impressed, too, with chia's large amount of fiber and natural antioxidants. Their conclusion: "The potential of this seed, for health and nutrition, [is] of a very remarkable level." Remarkable, indeed!

CHIA NUTRITION FACTS AT A GLANCE	
Nutrient	**Per 1 ounce (about 2 tablespoons)**
Calories	138
Protein	4.7 g
Fat	8.7 g
Carbohydrate	11.9 g
Fiber	9.8 g
Omega-3s	5.1 g
Omega-6s	1.6 g
Omega-9s	0.6 g
Calcium	179 mg
Iron	2.2 mg
Magnesium	95 mg
Phosphorus	244 mg
Potassium	115 mg
Zinc	1.3 mg
Copper	0.26 mg
Vitamin C	0.5 mg
Thiamin	0.177 mg
Riboflavin	.05 mg
Niacin	2.5 mg
Folate	14 μg
Vitamin A	15 IU
Vitamin E	.14 mg

Source: U.S. Department of Agriculture (USDA) National Nutrient Database for Standard Reference.

Omega-3s

Maybe when you hear the term *omega-3s*, you think "fish." That's natural: seafood is an excellent source of omega-3s, and most studies use fish oil to test the benefits of omega-3s. But fish is in no way the *only* source of omega-3s, so if you never, or only rarely, eat fish, don't worry—chia to the rescue! (And even if you do eat fish, it's nice to know there are alternatives. I mean, just how much salmon can one person eat?)

Omega-3s are "essential fatty acids"—nutrition lingo that means your body cannot make them itself. These fatty acids are made up of chains of carbon atoms: the omega-3 fatty acid in plants (alpha-linolenic acid, ALA), is made up of short-chain fats; the omega-3 fatty acids in fish oils (eicosapentaenoic acid, EPA, and docosahexaenoic acid, DHA), are made up of long-chain fats. Your body can use EPA and DHA right away. ALA, on the other hand, requires a little more work before you can fully benefit from it: your body must convert it to EPA and DHA

Estimates on how much ALA gets converted vary. For a while, it was assumed that the conversion rate was fairly low (5 to 10 percent); now, though, experts are beginning to think that the conversion rate may be better than originally thought. In Great Britain, researchers set out to see the differences in omega-3 levels between people who ate meat and fish, people who ate meat but *not* fish, vegetarians, and vegans. One of the study goals was to understand how the many people who don't eat fish can still get the omega-3s they need for good health. The study was also motivated by the fact that the supply of wild fish is threatened and many of the fish being served up these days are compromised by mercury and other pollutants (see page 74 for more on fish safety).

It was a big study that included more than fourteen thousand men and women who kept seven-day food diaries, allowing the researchers to monitor their intake of omega-3s. Blood levels of omega-3s were tested in a subset of nearly five thousand of the participants. The results showed that the non–fish eaters consumed from 20 to 43 percent fewer omega-3 fatty acids than the fish eaters; however, the blood tests showed that the non–fish eaters were closer in EPA/DHA status to the fish eaters than might be expected. This indicated that the non–fish eaters were converting ALA at a rate higher than previous statistics had suggested. The researchers also found that women (at least women of reproductive age) had higher rates of ALA conversion then men, a phenomenon—possibly due to effects of estrogen—shown in many other studies as well.

So that's good news! And as an added bonus, ALA seems to have some benefits of its own. In 2005, data from the Nurses' Health Study—one of the largest and most important investigations into women's health—showed that a diet rich in ALA significantly reduced the risk of sudden cardiac death. This reinforces the results of a study that tested out the effects of the Indo-Mediterranean diet, which is high in ALA. The subjects, one thousand people at risk for coronary heart disease, were divided up into two groups: one consumed a typical low-cholesterol diet and the other the Indo-Mediterranean, ALA-rich diet. After two years, the ALA group had significantly lowered rates of heart attacks and death due to cardiac events.

The Benefits of Omega-3s

You hear so much about omega-3s these days, but with little mention of the fact that plants can be a good source of these important nutrients. I hope the ascent of chia will help change the dialogue: these seeds should be better known for adding valuable omega-3 fats to the diet.

Instead of asking what benefits omega-3s offer, you might ask what benefits these fatty acids *don't* supply. William Sears, MD, the eminent pediatrician and health advocate, has called omega-3s the "head-to-toe healing nutrient," and I think it's the perfect description—research shows that omega-3s can have an effect on everything from anxiety to heart arrhythmias, and just about everything in between. That's likely because omega-3s have both protective *and* therapeutic powers. Not only can they help you dodge a laundry list of diseases, they can help restore your health if you already have symptoms.

Here are just some of the good things omega-3s can do for you:

- **Omega-3s give you a healthier heart.** Regular intake of omega-3s lowers cholesterol, triglycerides, blood pressure, and other markers of cardiovascular disease.

- **Omega-3s lower your risk of cancer.** Researchers are still looking into the association between omega-3s and reduced cancer risk, but the science looks promising, particularly in regard to breast cancer. In the laboratory at least, omega-3s can inhibit breast tumors, and some epidemiological studies have shown that women with higher intakes of omega-3s have lower rates of the disease.

- **Omega-3s reduce symptoms of autoimmune disease.** Having not had a trace of autoimmune problems since I began eating chia, this is one effect of omega-3s that I can personally vouch for. Autoimmune diseases—and there are a wide variety of them—occur when your immune system inexplicably attacks healthy cells, causing an array of symptoms such as fatigue, muscle aches, skin eruptions, and hair loss. Having one of these diseases can be awful; they're often debilitating and can be life threatening. But omega-3s can help. Several studies have shown that omega-3s reduce joint pain and swelling in people who have rheumatoid arthritis. An investigation into the effects of omega-3s on lupus also turned up positive results. Conducted in Ireland, the 2008 study looked at what happened when lupus sufferers received omega-3 supplements, then compared them to people who also had the disease but received placebos for the study's duration. At the end of twenty-four weeks, the omega-3 group had reduced disease activity in their skin and joints, while the participants who got a placebo had no improvements. You can see why I couldn't get these mighty seeds into my diet fast enough!

THE ANTI-INFLAMMATORY EFFECT OF OMEGA-3S

Inflammation, experts suspect, is the culprit behind a lot of diseases, including heart disease, Alzheimer's disease, and diabetes. According to the American Autoimmune Related Diseases Association, there's also some suggestion that inflammation can provoke autoimmune reactions in people with a genetic predisposition for the disorders. Autoimmune disorders themselves cause inflammation, too, which can damage tissue and lead to some of the diseases' more severe symptoms, such as swelling in the joints of rheumatoid arthritis sufferers.

But here again, omega-3s are a star: They can get in there and inhibit the formation of hormones that cause inflammation, helping to stop the damage. In 2012, Ohio State University researchers put the anti-inflammatory capability of omega-3s to the test by giving 138 men and women either a placebo or a dose of the healthy fatty acids—either 2.5 or 1.25 grams of omega-3s per day. The people in the study were all middle-aged and overweight, but otherwise healthy (inflammation can be a side effect of excess body fat, which made the subjects good study candidates). After four months of supplementation, both groups receiving the omega-3s had significantly lower levels of inflammation markers in their blood, while the placebo group showed no difference in the same markers.

- **Omega-3s keep your brain in good working order.** Omega-3s help keep brain cell membranes soft and flexible and improve actions—like connections between brain cells—that enable you to think more quickly and remember more. So it's not surprising that when researchers looked at dietary information from more than seventeen thousand people, they found that those who ate a diet rich in omega-3 fatty acids—as well as low in saturated fats, meat, and dairy foods—had better memory function and better thinking ability.

- **Omega-3s do about a hundred other things.** I exaggerate. It's not a hundred, but the number of possible perks from omega-3s is really astounding. Not only are omega-3s showing promise in soothing depression and lessening symptoms of attention deficit hyperactivity disorder (ADHD) and attention deficit disorder (ADD), they may also help you control your appetite, slow aging, reduce damage from sunburn, and relieve skin conditions such as eczema, psoriasis, and dermatitis. Some research also suggests that omega-3s can cool hot flashes, reduce the risk of macular degeneration, and lessen menstrual pain.

||||||||||||||||||||||||||||||||||||||||||||||||||||||||||||||||||||||||||||||||||||||||||||||||||||||||||||||||||||||||||||

RAMP UP OMEGA-3S / SCALE BACK OMEGA-6S

When you round up the research and look at our Western diet, it's clear: we need more omega-3s! But that's not all. According to many experts, we also need to *reduce* our omega-6 intake. Like omega-3s, omega-6s are essential fatty acids that the body cannot produce on its own. Both are important for proper body functions, such as maintaining bone health and producing hormones. (There is another group of omegas, omega-9s, which the body needs but can make on its own.) However, whereas omega-3s are anti-inflammatory, omega-6s *generate* inflammation. What's more, omega-3s have to compete with omega-6s for vital enzymes, and omega-3s generally lose out, diminishing the benefits you get from them. Omega-6s also interfere with the conversion of ALA to EPA and DHA (see pages 20–21 for an explanation of the conversion process), reducing it by as much as 40 to 50 percent. That's a lot!

The typical American diet has roughly eleven to thirty times more omega-6s than omega-3s, a very lopsided ratio, especially when you compare it with diets in other cultures: in Japan, where the incidence of heart disease and cancer is relatively low, the ratio is closer to 2 to 1. Not all health experts agree that Americans need to lower their omega-6 intake, but some evidence certainly seems to suggest the value of striving for a better omega-3/omega-6 balance. For example, a 2013 Ohio State University study found that as the ratio of omega-6s to omega-3s (from both fish and plant sources) decreased, so did the risk of hip fractures in older women. And when University of California at Los Angeles researchers compared the breast tissue of seventy-three women with breast cancer with that of seventy-four women without breast cancer, the breast adipose (fat) tissue of the women with cancer had higher levels of omega-6s and lower levels of omega-3s. The 2002 study also showed that the reverse was true of the women without cancer, leading the researchers to conclude that omega-6s might contribute to breast cancer, while omega-3s might have a protective effect.

Most fats have some omega-6s, even chia. What you want to limit, though, are fats with a heavy ratio of omega-6s to omega-3s. With that in mind, moderate your consumption of the following:

Corn oil
Safflower oil
Processed foods and snacks
Sunflower oil
Cottonseed oil
Soybean oil
Peanut oil
Sesame oil
Grapeseed oil

SEEDS OF WISDOM

· ·

Let food be thy medicine and medicine be thy food.

—HIPPOCRATES, *ancient Greek physician*

How Much Omega-3s Do You Need?

Two tablespoons (28 grams) of chia seeds have a whopping 5.1 grams of omega-3s, the highest level of total omega-3 fatty acids of any plant source. That will get you going in the morning! The U.S. Department of Agriculture's recommended dietary allowance (RDA) for alpha-linolenic acid, the kind of omega-3s in chia, is 1.1 grams for women and 1.6 grams for men, so you can see that, if you're following the *Chia Vitality* eating plan, you don't have to even think about how you're going to get enough omega-3s—it's all there and then some. You'll see what I mean when you sample the yummy *Chia Vitality* recipes in chapter 9 and start tossing chia into (almost) everything. It will all add up to a more energetic, disease-resistant, and vibrant you!

ATHLETE ALERT: NEXT TIME, CONSIDER CHIA LOADING

Carbohydrate loading is a time-honored practice of athletes gearing up for endurance exercise sessions. Could chia do the same job? The Human Performance Laboratory at the University of Alabama, Auburn, decided to find out. Researchers recruited six endurance athletes and had them follow a loading protocol using either a chia beverage mixed 50/50 with a traditional sports drink or a traditional sports drink alone for two days before an endurance test. The test, a one-hour run on a treadmill, was followed by a 10K time trial on a track. A few weeks later, the athletes switched drinks and repeated the steps.

When the results were all in, both protocols affected performance equally well, but the athletes who drank the chia-spiked sports drink had a few advantages: using chia allowed them to cut the amount of sports drink in half, so they took in less sugar than the 100 percent sports drink group—and got some omega-3 fatty acids, fiber, and protein in the bargain. If you're going to carb-load for energy, why not get the most nutrients you can?

Protein

When you talk about protein, what you're really talking about is a collection of amino acids, organic compounds that add up to form protein. Like certain omega-3s, some amino acids are "essential"—of the twenty or so that exist, your body cannot make nine of them, so it's critical that you get them through food. That's why the quality of the protein you eat is so important.

Your best sources are what are known as "complete proteins," meaning that they have all nine of the essential amino acids. Beef, pork, poultry, fish, eggs, and dairy products usually get top billing in the complete-protein show, but guess what? Chia is an excellent source of complete protein! Very few vegetable sources of amino acids are complete proteins. And the quality—judged by the proportions of amino acids in a food—is high: "higher than that of some cereals and other oilseeds," says food scientist Octavio Paredes-López, PhD, leader of the 2013 CINVESTAV chia study mentioned on page 18. Paredes-López also found that not only is the quality of protein high in chia seeds; so is the quantity: at 19 to 23 percent of their makeup, the amount of protein in chia is similar to that in lentils and chickpeas, other good sources of vegetarian protein, and higher than that in wheat, corn, rice, oats, and barley. And gram for gram, chia has more than twice the protein of tofu.

The Benefits of Protein

I asked Professor Paredes-López why protein is so important, and he put it very succinctly: "Proteins provide the structure for all living things—every organism, from the largest animal to the tiniest microbe, is composed of protein." Every metabolic reaction in your body, including DNA replication, and every response to potential trouble (like bacteria) involves protein. Protein, in short, is a vital player in every chemical process that sustains your life.

It also affects your *quality* of life, and one of the ways it does that is by helping you to stay strong. That's particularly true as you get older. You need protein to make muscle and to keep muscle from disappearing as you age (especially if you aren't physically active—remember the old "use or lose it" adage). By countering muscle loss, protein also helps you maintain a healthier weight: muscle tissue is ravenous for calories, so the more of it you have, the more calories you burn each day.

Protein also has something else going for it: it's extremely satisfying. That may have something to do with the fact that high-protein foods are slow to move out of your stomach and cause only small, gradual increases in blood sugar. When blood sugar rises rapidly, it's followed by a big dip that drives up your appetite. Small increases, on the other hand, help you avoid that desperate "I have to eat now!" feeling.

Many studies have shown that people eat less and stay fuller longer when their diet contains higher levels of protein. Even consuming a high-protein snack can help keep your appetite under control. Researchers at the University of Missouri have investigated the power of protein numerous times, including in a small but telling 2013 study that looked at how eating low-, moderate-, or high-protein snacks would influence subsequent eating behavior in a group of volunteers. For four days, fifteen young women randomly consumed 160-calorie portions of yogurt that contained one of the three levels of protein or no snack at all. The researchers then measured how full the women felt every thirty minutes and documented how long they went before requesting dinner. The high-protein yogurt led to reduced hunger and increased fullness and allowed the women to go longer before desiring to eat again.

How Much Protein Do You Need?

There's no need to load up on protein; even if you don't dive into a big steak every night, you probably get enough, because, in general, you need just 0.8 grams of protein per two pounds of body weight. If you weigh 130 pounds, that's 52 grams—about the equivalent of a chicken breast (30g), one cup of brown rice (5g), a few almonds (2g), and one cup of black beans (15g). However, rather than concentrating on how *much* protein you need, focus on the *kind* of protein you're getting. That steak I just mentioned? It gives you plenty of protein, but you get a lot of unhealthy saturated fat in the bargain. In fact, high intake of animal protein is linked to an increased risk of cancer and heart disease. So get your protein from chia and other sources that don't come with lots of damaging baggage in tow.

The *Chia Vitality* meal plan provides all the high-quality protein you require each day to feel satisfied and thrive. When you're not following the plan, keep your average needs as determined by the 0.8-gram-per-two-pounds formula in mind as well as the fact that it's an average recommendation; your body's needs change depending on what you're doing. For instance, exercise breaks down muscle and builds it back up again, which means you may need a little more protein to do the job. So if you're an avid endurance athlete—meaning you engage in long (two to five hours), fairly high-intensity bouts of exercise—you may need up to 50 percent more protein. In that case, use 0.6 gram of protein per pound of body weight to calculate your needs.

HOW HEALTHY PROTEIN SOURCES STACK UP			
Food	**Serving Size**	**Protein (grams)**	
Chia	2 tablespoons (28 g)	4.7	Seeds
Flaxseeds	2 tablespoons (28 g)	5.1	
Sunflower seeds	2 tablespoons (28 g)	5.8	
Pepitas (pumpkin seeds)	2 tablespoons (28 g)	5.2	
Almonds	1 ounce (about 22 nuts)	6	Nuts
Walnuts	1 ounce (about 14 halves)	4.3	
Cashews	1 ounce (about 17 nuts)	4.3	
Pecans	1 ounce (about 19 nuts)	2.6	
Pistachios	1 ounce (about 49 nuts)	5.9	
Almond butter	2 tablespoons (28 g)	5.9	Nut Butters
Peanut butter	2 tablespoons (28 g)	7	
Soy milk	1 cup	7	Milks
Almond milk	1 cup	1	
Hemp milk	1 cup	5	
Rice milk	1 cup	0.67	
Soybeans (edamame)	1 cup	22	Beans and Legumes
Black beans	1 cup	15.2	
Pinto beans	1 cup	15.4	
Lentils	1 cup	17.9	
Brown rice	1 cup	5	
Quinoa	1 cup	8.1	
Bulgur	1 cup	5.6	
Tofu, firm	½ cup	10.3	Tofu
Tofu, silken	½ cup	8.1	

Eggs	1 large	6.3	Animal Sources
Chicken breast (skinless)	3 ounces	26.4	
Salmon	3 ounces	23.3	
Tuna, canned	3 ounces	20.1	
Turkey, deli sliced	3 ounces	19.5	
Goat cheese, soft	1 ounce	5.2	Dairy
Parmesan cheese	2 tablespoons	3.8	
Yogurt, fruit flavored, nonfat	1 cup	10.8	
Greek yogurt, plain, nonfat	1 cup	23	
1% milk	1 cup	8.2	
Asparagus	1 cup (cooked)	4.3	Vegetables
Broccoli	1 cup (cooked)	3.7	
Spinach	1 cup (cooked)	5.3	
Kale	1 cup (raw)	2.9	

Source: U.S. Department of Agriculture (USDA) National Nutrient Database for Standard Reference.

Fiber

Some nutrients go about their jobs surreptitiously. Antioxidants, for instance. You might not feel their beneficial effects in any tangible way. Fiber's effects, though, are pretty immediate. You know it's working!

Dietary fiber is made up of plant compounds that largely go undigested by the body. There are two types of fiber, soluble and insoluble, and you need them both. Soluble dissolves in water; insoluble fiber does not. These physical characteristics allow fiber to do different things as they move through your system. When soluble fiber dissolves in the intestines, it forms a sticky gel that slows digestion and also grabs cholesterol, whisking it out of the body and making it less available to gum up your arteries. Insoluble fiber absorbs water and expands, helping to make you feel full and keep you "regular," quickly sweeping the harmful by-products of digestion out of your system.

Most of chia's fiber is insoluble, but it has soluble fiber, too. In fact, you can actually see it: when chia seeds get wet, they produce what's called mucilage—a sticky soluble-fiber gel that's clear and actually has a nice mouth feel. Some people have compared it to Jell-O, but it's a little less viscous. The gel might seem like a funny novelty at first, but as you'll see when you hit the recipes section, in addition to its health benefits, the gel has some unique culinary properties that make it great to cook with. You can, for instance, use it to make healthy puddings, and it adds body to salad dressings and smoothies.

Trying to figure out whether you're getting enough of both kinds of fiber could make you crazy, and the truth is, your total fiber intake is what matters most. What's important to know about chia is that the seeds are made up of about 33 percent fiber—superior to other good sources of fiber, such as flaxseeds (22 percent), barley (17 percent), corn (13 percent), wheat (12 percent), and soybeans (15 percent).

The Benefits of Fiber

The most obvious of fiber's benefits are those involving your gastrointestinal tract. Most fiber passes through the digestive system, helping to prevent constipation and the disease diverticulitis, an inflammation of the intestine. Because fiber is bulky and slows digestion, it can make you feel full—one reason people who eat a lot of fiber tend to carry around less body fat than people who eat little fiber. Fiber-rich foods also tend to take a longer time to chew (think apples versus ice cream), an experience that makes you less likely to gobble your food down and gives your brain time to get the message that you're full.

Fiber has also been associated with lowering the risk of some of our worst ills. It protects against cardiovascular disease by reducing blood pressure and LDL (low-density lipoprotein), or "bad," cholesterol. Some research also suggests that eating a diet high in fiber will lower your risk of both stroke and diabetes—all the more reason to pack more chia into your day.

SEEDS OF KNOWLEDGE

. . . .

GLUTEN-FREE FIBER

It's happening all over: people who were once big bread and pasta eaters are developing sensitivities to gluten, a protein found in wheat and some of its relatives, such as barley, rye, and spelt. If you've always gotten most of your fiber from wheat, giving it up can put a big dent in your intake—but not if you're eating chia. Chia has lots of fiber and not a smidgen of gluten. It's completely gluten free. Of course, there are lots of gluten-free products on the market now and other naturally gluten-free grains and seeds to choose from (such as rice, quinoa, and some oats), but it's nice to know you don't have to forsake chia to stay gluten free and that it can help fill in any fiber gaps in your diet.

How Much Fiber Do You Need?

For every 2 tablespoons of chia you eat, you get about 10 grams of fiber. That's huge! For comparison, a half cup of cooked black beans has 8 grams of fiber; a slice of whole wheat bread, 3 grams; a cup of cooked brown rice, 2 grams; an apple, 4 grams; a half cup of broccoli, 2 grams. Chia is truly a fiber superstar, especially when you consider how close it gets you to your daily requirements. The recommended dietary allowance (RDA) for women under the age of fifty-one is 25 grams of fiber per day (21 grams if you're over age fifty-one). Men under the age of fifty-one should get 38 grams of fiber per day (30 grams if you're over age fifty-one). That's a big step up if you've only been getting as much fiber as most Americans do—a paltry 15 grams—but chia is going to make it easy for you to meet the RDA.

SEEDS OF WISDOM
· ·

If we are creating ourselves all the time, then it is never too late to begin creating the bodies we want instead of the ones we mistakenly assume we are stuck with.

—DEEPAK CHOPRA, *physician and author*

Antioxidants

It wasn't that long ago that no one had heard of antioxidants. Now people are tossing off the word as if they've known it since preschool (*Can you believe how many antioxidants that smoothie has?*). But not everyone knows exactly what antioxidants are or why they are so important. In case you're among the uninitiated (and don't feel bad if you are—this stuff gets complicated!), here's a little antioxidant primer.

To understand antioxidants, it helps to first understand free radicals. You create free radicals—molecules that are missing critical electrons—just through the daily process of living. Burning fats and carbohydrates, for instance, creates free radicals. Outside factors, too, can increase the production of free radicals. Unhealthy foods, polluted air, alcohol, cigarette smoke, pollutants, and sun exposure all generate them; even healthy things like exercise can speed up the creation of these errant molecules.

The trouble with free radicals is that, in need of electrons, they proceed to steal them from other places in the body, including DNA, proteins, and cell membranes. Without those electrons, the healthy cells cease to function properly and may even die. Over time, this can wreak havoc on the natural order within the body and cause real damage: cancer, heart disease, and memory loss are all associated with the harm done by free radicals. Dermatologists place a lot of the blame for lines and wrinkles on free radicals, believing that they can also speed up the appearance of aging.

The white knights in all this are antioxidants. These substances save the day by deactivating the marauding free radicals, preventing them from stealing electrons and from leaving destruction in their wake. While the body manufactures some antioxidants on its own, getting more through food in the form of phytochemicals is believed to markedly ratchet up the body's defense system. There are many different kinds of antioxidants, and they work in different ways as well as synergistically, so you need a variety of them. That's one reason you can't just load up on vitamin E supplements or eat a bushel of carrots for its beta-carotene (both E and beta-carotene are important antioxidants) and expect to have your health improve.

The Benefits of Antioxidants

Here's a rundown of the most prominent antioxidants in chia and how they can improve your health.

- **Quercetin**—This antioxidant is in the flavonoid category, a group of antioxidants that not only have free-radical-fighting powers but are also anti-inflammatory and antiallergic. Some laboratory studies have shown that quercetin can disable cancer cells, and it may help prevent heart disease. Interestingly, it's conceivable that quercetin also has something to do with chia's power to ramp up stamina. A 2009 University of South Carolina study found that quercetin increases endurance by 13.2 percent and aerobic fitness by 3.9 percent.

- **Chlorogenic acid**— Also found in coffee, cholorogenic acid is believed to have anticancer properties and may also help reduce the risk of type 2 diabetes by positively affecting blood sugar. Some research in animals has also shown that this antioxidant increases fat burning, which may help lower body weight. I know you appreciate that!

- **Caffeic acid**—Caffeic acid is being looked at for its potential ability to inhibit growth of cancer cells and viruses and for its possible antidiabetic properties. One study (in rats) found that it may help increase exercise endurance.

- **Kaempferol**—The list of "antis" for this flavonoid is long: antioxidant, anti-inflammatory, anticancer, anti–cardiovascular disease, antidiabetic, anti-osteoporotic. Of particular note: studies have found associations with kaempferol intake and reduced risk of pancreatic and lung cancers.

SEEDS OF KNOWLEDGE

NO PRESERVATIVES NEEDED

Just as antioxidants prevent oxidation in your body, they prevent oxidation in plants. That's why chia is so shelf stable—it can last for years in a cool, dry place. Whole chia seeds have even been found buried in graves that were hundreds of years old (though I wouldn't advise eating them!).

How Much Antioxidants Do You Need?

If only we knew! There are dietary recommendations for certain antioxidants like vitamins A, C, and E, but not for the type of phytochemicals found in chia. We do know, though, that it's best to get your antioxidants through foods, not supplements, and that you can ensure getting optimal amounts by eating ample amounts of fruits, vegetables, whole grains, and seeds. When you get your antioxidants through food, there's little chance of getting too many: in this case, more antioxidant foods (but not antioxidant supplements) is more.

Another way to ensure you get maximal amounts of antioxidants is to choose ones—like chia—that contain an array of those beneficial compounds. You'll also get more antioxidants if you stick to unprocessed, unadulterated *whole* foods: processed foods generally lose something as they're being prepared for packaging, and often that something is antioxidants.

OTHER CHIA ATTRIBUTES

Minuscule though it may be, a chia seed is stuffed with the vitamins and minerals your body needs to thrive. Especially worth a mention: Two tablespoons of chia seeds provide 12 percent of a day's requirement of calcium and 8 percent of daily needs for iron. Chia is also rich in copper and boasts vitamin E, niacin, folate, magnesium, manganese, potassium, selenium, and zinc. I know! I can't believe there's all that stashed inside those minuscule seeds.

So far, there haven't been many studies that look specifically at the benefits of chia, but some research is starting to appear (and expect to see more on the way). For instance, in a 2007 study, researchers at the Risk Factor Modification Centre, St. Michael's Hospital in Toronto, Canada, and a group at the University of Toronto tested out a chia-supplemented diet on people with diabetes to see if chia would lower some of the cardiovascular risks caused by the disease. The twenty men and women in the study spent twelve weeks consuming either 37 grams of Salba—a name-brand form of chia—or wheat bran. They then had several "wash-out" weeks to get their systems back to normal, after which they switched: those who had wheat bran the first time crossed over to chia and vice versa. At the end of the study, the chia eaters had lower systolic blood pressure and lower levels of CRP (C-reactive protein), a marker of inflammation. Chia did reduce their risk of heart disease—just as the researchers had hoped.

CHIA FOR HEARTBURN

For years, my husband, Lance, suffered from heartburn. It was awful, and he was frequently taking prescription drugs to minimize the symptoms. Shortly after I discovered chia, I suggested that he try chia seeds as a heartburn remedy. Not only did it work, he's been free and clear of acid reflux ever since.

The most likely reason is that the seeds, which are like a sponge, absorb excess acid in the stomach. Lance takes one tablespoon of dry chia in the morning with a sip of water and it seems to do the trick. Some people wash the dry chia down with one sip, then drink a cup of water about five minutes later. Both approaches seem to work.

LOSING WEIGHT WITH CHIA

You don't have to be skinny to be full of life and vitality. There's no doubt, though, that being a healthy weight can help you live longer and help you stay vibrant for a longer stretch of time. And weight doesn't just affect your longevity; it affects your quality of life. Being a healthy weight helps you move with ease and feel fitter so that you can accomplish all those things you want to accomplish. Part of having vitality is getting out there and doing stuff!

Chia possesses many attributes that can help with weight loss. Most notably, the seeds absorb twelve times their weight—yes, that's right *twelve times*!—taking up space in your stomach that you might otherwise fill with excess calories. When Canadian researchers gave twenty people varying doses (7, 15, and 24 grams) of either ground or whole chia baked into bread, they stayed fuller longer than when they ate bread without the seeds. The chia also helped lower their postmeal blood sugar, a benefit that can help reduce the risk of diabetes.

Chia may also promote weight loss by lowering the number

of calories you absorb (thank the fiber for that neat trick). On its own, chia has only 70 calories per tablespoon, and its macronutrient makeup—lots of satiating protein, lots of satiating fiber—is of the most hunger-quenching kind. The fact that the seeds also help keep blood sugar steady means you won't have those roller-coaster highs and lows that can make you want to tear open a bag of potato chips and eat until that loopy feeling goes away.

I think it goes without saying that you can't exist on a diet of doughnuts and soda with a side of chia and expect the numbers on your scale to drop in any meaningful way. That's too much heavy lifting even for this superseed—or any superfood, for that matter. Still, chia's effect on appetite and blood sugar can make following a healthy, lower-calorie diet easier, and that can result in pounds dropping off. It bears mentioning, too, that by making you feel more vital and alive, chia increases the energy you have to say no to junk and yes to healthy whole foods (think about how easy it is to settle for fast food and other trashy conveniences when you're tired). Chia gives you more energy to exercise, too, and that can only help you shave off pounds.

As you'll see when you reach the 30-day *Chia Vitality* meal plan, it's not a weight loss diet per se. But it's set up so you can adjust the calories to shed pounds if you want to. The optional three-day cleanse, beginning on page 76, can help you kick-start weight loss if that's one of your goals. There are only so many pounds you can safely drop in three days' time, but the cleanse can help you get motivated to take further steps to slim down.

DR. OZ'S CHIA EXPERIMENT

Not too long ago, Mehmet Oz, MD, better known simply as Dr. Oz, conducted an interesting little experiment on his television show. I should say first that Dr. Oz is a big chia lover. Like me, he's a true believer! With this experiment, he set out to prove what he knew to be true: that chia seeds can keep you full all day.

To test his hypothesis, Dr. Oz had two self-described stress eaters—one who said she couldn't go more than a few hours without chocolate and another who said that when she was stressed she'd go for things like cheese and crackers—swap their usual snacking habits for a regimen of two tablespoons of chia stirred into water after breakfast and again after lunch. He then had the women on his show to share their results. You could have knocked both of them over with a feather! They were absolutely shocked at how their cravings ceased and how full they felt for the remainder of the day. Both said they ate very little dinner on their chia regimen day.

This was only a one-day study—it's not going to make it into the annals of science. But thank you, Dr. Oz! His little experiment totally jibes with what I hear about chia all the time.

Even though many health experts are already singing the praises of chia, I feel we've just scratched the surface. Once more research on chia's benefits gets under way, I believe we're going to hear a lot more about all that chia can do for our well-being. But no need to wait! We already know that chia brings enormous amounts of nutrients to the table. In the next chapter I'll tell you all you need to know to harness the power of this superseed.

3

. . . .

SEEDS OF
A CHANGED DIET

One of the qualities I associate with vitality is enthusiasm. When you're excited about something, it's like taking a happy pill—it can positively change the tenor of your day, your week, your life! My enthusiasm for chia, which knows no bounds (as if you hadn't noticed), led me in directions I could never have imagined. I'm living proof of the amazing things that can happen when you latch on to something you love.

Typically, all that love and enthusiasm triggers a desire for knowledge. This seems particularly true—in health-conscious people at least—when the object of interest is a food. You want to know everything about it. That's how I felt about chia, though at first all I could think about was *How can I get more of this great stuff?* I realized I needed to ask some more probing questions, such as, Where does chia come from? Who grows it? What's the best way to consume it? What's hype, and what's the real deal? It's just like meeting the love of your life. You can't get enough of the person in the early days, but at some point you've got to gather all the information you need to ensure that what began as a lovely infatuation will turn into an enduring relationship.

This chapter is designed to help you become part of the chia cognoscenti—those of us who not only consume chia with gusto but know the best ways to source it, use it, and integrate it into a vitality-promoting diet. I'll fill you in on everything from buying the seeds

41

to choosing among the different chia products to incorporating them into your kitchen. I'm going to weigh in, too, on filling your pantry and fridge with the other foods that round out the *Chia Vitality* diet.

By now, you've probably already seen chia in the grocery store and have even tried it or are eating it regularly. But, chia novice or old hand, I think you'll find this chapter an enlightening guide to stocking your kitchen well—and in a way that's good for both you and the planet.

FROM STALK TO SUPERMARKET

Despite its having been around for thousands of years, chia is relatively new to most of us. And as a dietary staple, the story of chia is still evolving. In the near future, expect to see more of this diminutive dynamo on your store shelves and in varying guises. That's one reason I want to not only share my love of chia with you but turn you into a chia expert! The better acquainted you are with the seeds, the more use you'll get out of them and the savvier you'll be about shopping for chia. Anything that attains superfood status is ripe for exploitation—in other words, you're probably going to begin seeing chia in foods that aren't really as healthful as their manufacturers advertise—so we've all got to be smart about how we source these magnificent seeds.

WHERE DOES CHIA COME FROM?

If you're anything like me, you like to know how your food was grown and where it comes from. So picture, if you will, fields of tall, spiky stalks with beautiful purple flowers. In their full-grown glory, chia plants actually look very different from the little green sprouts you see on Chia Pets. As classified by botanists, chia—*Salvia hispanica*—is technically an herb, part of the mint family (Lamiaceae). And its seeds are, well, seeds. Like amaranth, quinoa, and buckwheat, which are also seeds, chia is often mistakenly called a grain. There's actually a slight botanical difference between the two. A seed is an ovule, similar to an egg after fertilization, while a grain is actually a small edible fruit.

Chia grows best in tropical or subtropical climates, so most of the seeds you'll find on the market come from far afield, primarily Mexico, Central and South America, and Australia. If you're an avid gardener, it's entirely possible to grow chia at home in warm weather. But if you're like most people, you'll probably be rooting around the supermarket shelves for chia rather than digging it up in your backyard.

So does it matter which producer or country your chia comes from? I don't think about *where* chia is grown so much as *how* it's grown: organically, please! I'll talk more about organic food beginning on page 58, but for now, suffice it to say that it's the one criterion I recommend sticking to as you shop for chia. Chia is inherently pest resistant, so many growers don't use pesticides, but they do use herbicides and synthetic fertilizers; therefore a good deal of chia is *not* organic. Look for the USDA Organic symbol on the package to be sure you're getting the cleanest product.

CHIA FOR YOUR SKIN

Just about the time chia started to explode on supermarket shelves, I began noticing it was showing up in the cosmetics aisle, too. And not only was chia (more specifically, chia oil) being incorporated into skin care products sold in natural foods stores, it was turning up in doctor-formulated serums and touted as the beauty secret of models and actresses. A friend visiting Japan sent me photos of rows of chia seed skin care products being sold at a popular cosmetics shop in Tokyo. No one is more on top of trends than the Japanese, so you know that if they're loving it over there, chia beauty has hit the big time!

As it happens, chia does almost as much for you on the outside as it does for you on the inside. Its perfect balance of omega-3s and omega-6s hydrates the skin and helps to keep moisture from escaping. One Korean study found that chia significantly improved the skin of patients with end-stage renal disease, a condition that turns the complexion superdry and itchy. Using a chia-based topical formulation for eight weeks, the participants in the study had better-hydrated skin and even lost some of the brownish patches that typify the disease. The researchers also tested the chia oil on people who didn't have the disease but had itchy eczema. Their skin improved, too.

When you look for chia cosmetics, use the same criteria you use for choosing foods: if the chia oil is at the end of a long ingredient list, the product probably doesn't offer much chia.

BUYING AND STORING CHIA

It used to be that anyone interested in chia had to really hunt the seeds down, traveling from one Mexican grocer to the next or digging them up in the odd prescient natural foods market. These days? I'm delighted to say we're living in a chia world. The number of companies now making seeds available has simply exploded. As you'd expect, natural food markets are still ground zero for chia; most continue to be well stocked. But, chances are, your neighborhood supermarket and even your local big-box store is selling chia in the health and wellness aisle now, too. Even Walmart sells chia. And it's available every which way. You can scoop it from the bulk bins (in natural foods stores), purchase it in small pouches, bring it home in recyclable tubs, and buy it in three-pound bags. If you live in a town where natural foods stores are sparse, you can purchase the seeds online directly from their producers, online grocers, and amazon.com. Google "organic chia seeds," and you'll have them at your door in no time.

Once you're in a chia state of mind, you're going to begin noticing that there's a flood of new chia-based products on the market.

Some that I've seen include chia tortillas, chia chips, chia popcorn, chia power bars, chia peanut butters, chia waffles, chia bread, and chia cereals. I told you we're living in a chia world! It's great to see the chia love spreading around, but—and here's where it gets sticky because obviously Mamma Chia is a purveyor of chia drinks and snacks, and I don't want to sound like I'm slamming the competition—not all chia products are created equal. Being in the food and beverage business has taught me a lot about the quality as well as the quantity of ingredients companies can opt to use in their products, and if there's one bit of wisdom I'd like to pass on, it's this: read the label closely. If "chia seeds" are among the last words you see on a long list of ingredients, chances are you're not getting much chia in the food you're buying. (The exception: if there are only three or four ingredients in a product, having chia at the end can still mean you're getting a good dose of seeds). Sometimes manufacturers throw in a very minimal amount of chia just so they can hop on the chia bandwagon. In some cases, it may not matter to you that a food has only a small portion of chia—consider it a bonus. But if you're counting on it to provide you with a significant amount of seeds, make sure the product delivers on its promise by checking the label.

It probably goes without saying (but I'll say it anyway) that chia foods should be held to the same standards you use to judge other foods you eat. When foods are processed, they're usually stripped of something, whether it's vitamins and minerals, phytochemicals, protein, fiber—or all of the above. So not only do you lose out on particular nutrients when you eat processed foods, the nutrients that are left may not function as well when their counterparts are removed. One reason experts believe that some nutrients don't seem to fulfill their promise when you isolate them and give them in the form of supplements is because their benefits are dependent on the interaction of other compounds. That is the magic of the synergy I talked about in chapter 1! So stripping away some of a food's basic elements may also be stripping away its power to protect and heal.

While you're checking the label for chia, also scrutinize the other ingredients. I personally cross off my list foods with ingredients that I can't pronounce or that seem better suited to a chemistry experiment than to something you are going to put into your body. I'm wary, too, of foods that rely on tons of sugar for their appeal or are rife with unhealthy fats (such as trans and saturated fats, the kind that raise cholesterol) or artificial flavorings. Out of respect for your body, eat defensively (see the sidebar "Defensive Dining: What You *Don't* Want to See on the Ingredients List," on page 58).

You'll save money—and be best equipped for this 30-day program—if you buy chia in bags of one or two pounds. Plus you can't go wrong by having a pretty big stash in your cupboard. One of the beauties of chia is that you don't have to worry about its going stale or rancid. That's unusual for a food with such a high oil content (by contrast, I keep nuts in the freezer because they go rancid so quickly). The antioxidants in chia that are so protective of your health also protect the seeds from deterioration. So thanks to its excellent nutritional profile, chia is so shelf stable it can last for years in a cool, dry place. Things change, though, when chia meets water; Chia Gel needs to be stored in the refrigerator and is best used within a few days (see page 51 to learn how to make Chia Gel). But the whole dry seeds are perfectly safe sitting in your pantry.

In my own kitchen, along with jarfuls in my cupboards—glass mason jars make perfect containers—I keep chia in two open bowls on my counter. These two dishes, which I bought on a trip to Japan, nestle together to form a beautiful yin-yang sign; I fill one dish with white chia, the other with black. Having them on the counter puts the seeds right in my path—the more I see them, the more I use them— and I love what the dishes represent. In Chinese philosophy, the merging of yin and yang—two opposite but complementary forces like dark and light, hot and cold, male and female, water and fire— symbolize interconnectedness and interdependency in the natural world. Bringing them together is thought to maintain the harmony of the universe. How beautiful is that?! And if I can extrapolate a bit, I think it's also a nice metaphor for what it means to live a full and

SEEDS OF WISDOM

· ·

We are indeed much more than what we eat, but what we eat can nevertheless help us to be much more than what we are.

—ADELLE DAVIS, *author and pioneering nutritionist*

vibrant life. We all have more than one side to us. My observation is that people with vitality are people who embrace who they are. They acknowledge the darkness, but they temper it with light. They savor the highs and accept the lows. They relish tranquility and even see the value in chaos. In other words, they take on the whole of the human experience. In a small way, I'm reminded of that every day when I look into my bowls of chia.

MAKING CHIA CHOICES

As I mentioned, I have both black and white chia in my kitchen. Nutritionally, there's no meaningful difference between the two, so I say follow your personal leanings. To me, it's often just a matter of aesthetics. The contrast of white seeds mixed into dark dishes can look very appealing, as can black seeds mixed into light. (Black chia seeds are actually a little closer to gray than to black.) Either one can also go undercover; you can barely see white seeds in light dishes or black seeds in dark ones. For instance, when I make dark berry chia drinks, I prefer to use black seeds; when I'm making coconut mango drinks, I'll use the white. Occasionally I'll use a mix of seeds, as in the Asian Pan-Seared Chia-Crusted Salmon with Spinach (page 176). Think about how the Japanese use white and black sesame seeds to add color and texture to food, then follow suit.

SEEDS OF KNOWLEDGE

NO AX TO GRIND:
WHOLE SEEDS DELIVER THE GOODS

One of the things I immediately loved about chia is that you don't have to grind it to get its whole package of goodness. You might hear otherwise—as controversies go, it's a mild one, but some people believe you *do* need to grind chia just as you do flaxseeds—but I still fall squarely in the whole-seed camp. One reason is that studies show that people eating whole-seed chia experience a rise in their omega-3 levels (as well as other benefits), which wouldn't happen if the nutrients weren't available to the digestive system. Other benefits bear out in research, too. For instance, in the study cited on page 38, both milled and whole chia equally helped people stay fuller longer and lowered their postmeal blood sugar. My own experience also tells me that whole chia is the whole enchilada: I was only using whole chia when my health recovered, and that's evidence enough for me!

Wayne Coates of the Office of Arid Land Studies at the University of Arizona in Tucson and an expert on chia also stands firmly on the side of whole seeds, and his own animal research bears it out. In one study, Coates and his colleague Ricardo Ayerza Jr. fed rats diets that contained either whole chia seeds, ground chia, chia oil, or no chia. All three of the chia diets contained equal amounts of omega-3s. At the end of thirty days, all the animals consuming chia in one form or another had higher levels of omega-3s than the animals consuming no chia. But those who ate the whole-seed chia had *significantly* higher levels. The researchers explained that, unlike flaxseed, which has a hard outer shell, chia seed has a soft shell, allowing our bodies to access all the goodies inside.

THE CHIA PANTRY

Most of the recipes in the *Chia Vitality* eating plan call for whole seeds or gel made from whole seeds. There are, though, varying forms of chia you'll likely encounter as you shop. As the chia expert you're on your way to becoming, you'll want to know the differences among them.

- **Whole Seeds**—These are your number one choice and the type of chia most of the *Chia Vitality* recipes call for. I prefer to eat foods with as little processing as possible, and chia is no exception. Since they're as healthy as ground chia, there's no reason not to eat whole chia seeds; for convenience and that fun mouth feel, whole seeds can't be beat.

- **Milled Seeds**—*Milled* is another word for *ground*. If you're not in love with the whole seeds' crunchiness or need a smoother ingredient for, say, baking, then opting for milled chia makes sense. Milled seeds can be more expensive, though; since the health benefits are the same as whole seeds, don't feel as though the more expensive option is necessarily the best one. Keep in mind that you can also grind chia yourself using a spice mill or a clean coffee grinder, blender, or food processor.

- **Chia Oil**—This mild-tasting oil can be used in salad dressings and baking, but it is too fragile to cook with otherwise. Unlike whole seeds, it doesn't have shelf endurance—you have to store it in the refrigerator. What you gain when you use chia oil is concentrated omega-3s (one tablespoon has 9 grams, while one tablespoon of seeds has about 2.5 grams); what you lose is fiber and protein (chia oil has none).

- **Chia Bran**—This slightly obscure form of chia is sort of the opposite of the oil: it provides plenty of chia's fiber and protein, but you lose a considerable amount of omega-3s. I don't think it makes much sense to separate chia seeds into parts—it's the whole package that makes them so amazing.

- **Chia Oil Supplements**—These soft-gel pills are packed with omega-3s and can be a vegetarian substitute for fish oils.

In my opinion, whole seeds are going to give you the best bang for your buck, but I do enjoy using milled chia and chia oil in some recipes, too. I encourage you to try different ways of integrating chia into your daily life and to let personal preference be your guide!

CHIA IN THE KITCHEN

Chia deserves all the acclaim it gets as a superfood. All those omega-3s, protein, fiber, and antioxidants—of course we sing its nutritional praises. But what often gets lost in all the expressions of admiration for the seeds' health prowess is one delicious little fact: chia is fun! On the one hand, you've got these dry little seeds that you can throw into just about anything for added crunch and texture. On the other hand, just add liquid and you've got a culinary tool for turning other foods velvety smooth. I've never had such a good time experimenting with a food. My kitchen has become a veritable chia lab, and I hope yours will, too!

The recipes for the *Chia Vitality* eating plan demonstrate how easy it is to cook with chia. Depending on what you're making, you can add chia before cooking (when you're making muffins or banana bread, for instance) or sprinkle the seeds in at the last minute (to rev up something like a stir-fry). Chia can transform no-cook dishes like salads and cereals from moderately beneficial to out-of-the-park healthy and give condiments a bump up in nutritional status—ketchup and mustard never looked so good. If you make your own frozen treats, scatter the seeds in an ice cream base as it churns, or stir a few tablespoons of

Chia Gel into juice and pour into a popsicle mold. Chia freezes well; you won't lose a scintilla of nutrients. (Mamma Chia drinks, by the way, make a great popsicle.)

SEEDS OF KNOWLEDGE
. . . .
CHIA GEL AS AN EGG SUBSTITUTE

If you have an egg allergy, are vegan, or are just a cook who likes to try new things (or you simply run out of eggs), Chia Gel is an ideal substitute. To replace a large egg, combine one tablespoon of chia seeds with three tablespoons of water. Whisk, then let sit until the gel forms, about fifteen minutes.

Once you begin working with chia, your mind will begin teeming with ideas on how to use it. If cooking isn't your thing, or you're in a phase when you're not spending much time in the kitchen, it's still easy to use chia. Add it to takeout food. Carry a little bag with you to restaurants so you can season your food with chia while dining out—it won't change the taste of your dish, but you can rest assured that you're giving an added nutritional punch to even the most decadent item on the menu. When you're sitting at your desk at work and start hitting the three o'clock wall, stir a tablespoon of chia seeds into a glass of water. It's a much better pick-me-up than the one you'll get from the vending machine. (You can drink the chia water quickly if you don't want it to gel, or you can stir it and allow a gel to form—it takes about fifteen minutes.) You can even do like the Tarahumara Indians do and snack on chia right from a little pouch.

I encourage you to be creative, to honor your own tastes, and to make adding chia to your food a habit. Think of it in the same way you do indispensable everyday accents like salt and pepper, only instead of adding a pinch of flavor, you'll be adding a dose of health and vitality to your food.

THROW AND GO:
20 EASY CHIA SEED ADD-INS

Chia Yogurt

Stir 2 teaspoons of chia seeds and 1 teaspoon of maple syrup (if the yogurt is unsweetened) into a half cup of nonfat Greek or Icelandic yogurt.

Chia Scrambled Eggs

Beat 2 eggs in a bowl, stir in 2 teaspoons of chia seeds, and cook as usual.

Chia Cereal

Sprinkle 2 teaspoons of chia seeds on top of hot or cold cereal.

Chia Sandwich

You can add chia to any sandwich. For a healthy variation on a peanut butter sandwich, slather almond butter on a slice of whole grain bread, sprinkle chia seeds to taste over the almond butter, then add the top slice of bread. Or simply add chia seeds to the condiment when making a turkey, ham, or veggie sandwich.

Chia Tuna or Egg Salad

Mix chia seeds into the prepared salad, using 1 teaspoon of seeds per serving.

Chia Refried Beans

Empty a can of refried beans into a pot, stir in 2 tablespoons of chia seeds, and warm over medium heat.

Chia Hummus

Stir 1 teaspoon of chia seeds per serving into any store-bought container of hummus.

Chia Rice

Cook rice as directed. Before serving, stir in $1/2$ teaspoon of white chia seeds per serving. Note that the seeds will be a little crunchy. If you prefer, you can cook the seeds with the rice, but you'll need to add about a tablespoon more water per teaspoon chia to the pot.

Chia Waffles

Stir 1 tablespoon of chia seeds into your favorite waffle batter, then cook as usual.

Chia Chocolate Chip Cookies

Stir 2 tablespoons of chia seeds into your favorite chocolate chip cookie batter, then bake as usual.

Chia Roasted Root Vegetables

Cut assorted root vegetables—parsnips, carrots, potatoes, sweet potatoes, beets—into 1-inch pieces; toss with olive oil and salt, then roast at 400°F until cooked through and caramelized. Add chia seeds to taste and toss again.

Chia Coleslaw

Sprinkle 1 teaspoon of chia seeds per serving into your favorite homemade or store-bought coleslaw.

Chia Pizza

Before serving, sprinkle a few pinches of chia seeds on top of your pizza, along with red pepper flakes or other favorite seasonings.

Chia Corn on the Cob

Brush a little olive oil on grilled or boiled corn on the cob, then roll the cobs in a plate of chia seeds.

Chia Quesadillas

Sprinkle shredded cheese on a tortilla; add any cooked (e.g., mushrooms) or shredded raw (e.g., zucchini) vegetables you like and 1 to 2 teaspoons of chia seeds. Top with a little more cheese and a second tortilla, then heat on a flat grill or pan.

Chia Tofu Scramble

Crumble a 14-ounce block of firm tofu, then season to taste. Sauté half a chopped onion in a little olive oil until soft, the add the tofu and 1 tablespoon of chia seeds. Sauté until warmed through, 3 to 5 minutes more.

Chia Muffins or Banana Bread

Add 1 tablespoon of chia seeds to your favorite muffin or banana bread batter and bake as usual.

Chia Vegetable Soup

Stir 1 tablespoon of chia seeds into your favorite recipe for vegetable soup, or 1 teaspoon per serving into canned soup.

Chia Lentils

Stir 2 teaspoons of chia seeds into 1 cup cooked lentils.

Chia Pasta

Stir 1 tablespoon of chia seeds into 12 to 16 ounces marinara sauce, warm, then toss with 1 pound of cooked pasta

STIR-CRAZY: MAKE A BOTTLED CONDIMENT OR DRESSING BETTER

An easy way to get more chia into your life is to add it in gel form to bottled ketchup, mustards, mayonnaise, relish, salsa, guacamole, chutney, and salad dressings. Cutting your condiments and dressings with chia will make them go further plus allow you to substantially increase their nutrients and cut their fat, calorie, and sugar contents.

Here's how to do it: Make a thick chia gel by adding 2 to 3 tablespoons of seeds to 1 cup of water, allowing it to sit for fifteen minutes. Place your condiment or dressing in a new container, then add the chia gel—about one-third gel to two-thirds condiment or dressing. The mixture will last 7 to 10 days in the refrigerator.

ROUNDING OUT THE REST OF YOUR DIET

There's a connection between vitality and a wholesome, nourishing diet that goes beyond the obvious. Eating well doesn't just keep you energized and preserve your health, it also gives you peace of mind—a key component of that more meaningful and purposeful life I keep talking about. When you're conscious (and conscientious) about where your food comes from and what it contains, you can not only take pleasure in knowing you're doing right by your body, you can also feel good about making an impact in the lives of other people as well.

In an intimate way, your food choices can influence the health of friends and family whom you feed. If you have kids, you're also modeling mindful behavior for them and giving them the message that eating is about more than answering the call of hunger. On a larger level, the food choices you make are also a vote for the kind of world you want to live in. If you're buying edibles that are produced humanely and safely, you're advocating for humane and safe practices and helping to further them along. If you're buying more whole foods and fewer processed ones, you're telling the marketplace that making healthy choices available is good business. You are one person, but when you add in your vote, these choices can benefit workers and eaters of all stripes.

Food is personal and food is political and I confess that it's often challenging to find the balance between the two. As I'm sure you've noticed by now, I hold strong beliefs about farming, food production, and wholesome eating. But I also *so* dislike food self-righteousness. There is nothing worse than having a holier-than-thou person looking down his or her nose at what you've got on your plate. To find that happy medium, I just follow my heart. I try to always honor and uplift both the soul of humanity and the soul of the planet by the choices I make in my personal and professional life. I do what's right for me, I share with others what I've learned, and I invest my time in organizations that further my values. Rather than pushing your ideals on someone else, it seems much more effective to simply show what conscious living can do for you. When people see you living a life that's filled with joy and vitality, they may be more inclined to follow your lead.

For this book, I've developed a diet that reflects both what many health experts consider to be the path to optimal health and what I've personally found leads to feeling vibrant and alive. It's built on predominately organic, non-GMO, and minimally processed whole foods—all with a sizable helping of chia, of course. If you're already eating this way, you may already know some of what follows, but at the risk of preaching to the choir, I'd like to state my case for why we all need to be choosy about the food we buy.

EAT WHOLE FOODS

"Whole foods" is not just a market! The term refers to foods in their most natural state, with all their nutrients intact. Brown rice is a whole food; white rice is not, because a lot of the nutrients, located in the bran and germ of the grain, have been tossed away to make it a smoother product. Likewise, whole wheat flour is a whole food; white flour is not. Chia seeds, both whole and ground, are a whole food.

There's a place for foods that have been processed to some degree. Think of olive oil; some fiber and other nutrients are lost in its production, but what you get is still delicious and nutritious and usable in far more ways than actual olives. Chia seed oil loses fiber and protein in the pressing process but has a considerable amount of omega-3s. So processing isn't all bad, and I'm not suggesting that you never eat foods that come in packages (I am in the food business, after all). Breads, cereals, fruit yogurts, condiments . . . they're all processed, but some brands are far better than others and don't cheat you of their ingredients' natural goodness. There are plenty of minimally and moderately processed foods that contain a large percentage of whole-some ingredients and which I wouldn't think twice about buying as long as they don't come bolstered with additives.

What I suggest, and what the *Chia Vitality* eating plan makes easy, is weighting your diet heavily toward whole foods. Eat clean whenever you can. That way, when you need to fill in with processed foods for convenience's sake (and, okay, for fun's sake, too—sometimes the pull of something junky is just way too hard to resist), you're still going to come out ahead. Remember, this isn't about perfection.

I also just want to note that it's easy to fall into the trap of think-ing that it's okay to eat everything that's a whole food without limit. Honey is a whole food. Salt is a whole food. A big block of Brie is a whole food. I think you get my drift—even unprocessed and mini-mally processed foods can undermine your vitality if you eat them in immoderate amounts. In particular, limit low and unprocessed foods that contain trans fats, known to raise cholesterol levels. Watch out, too, for high levels of saturated fats—meat and whole-fat dairy prod-ucts are the main sources—and go easy on foods made with whole ingredients that nonetheless drive up your sugar, fat, and salt intake. Potato chips or french fries made only from potatoes, salt, and a healthy oil might be considered whole foods, but they still fall in the junk food category, and, obviously, eating them to your heart's con-tent will catch up with you. That's especially true if you're eating them instead of other, more nutritious foods. Junk foods don't just junk up your system; they fill you up at the expense of healthier eating.

SEEDS OF WISDOM

When eating fruit, remember who planted the tree; when drinking water, remember who dug the well.

—VIETNAMESE PROVERB

When you do indulge, opt for products that have the least amount of processing, the fewest number of ingredients, and the most natural ingredients. I'd personally take a half cup of premium organic ice cream over two cups of fat-free ice cream made with fillers and a sugar substitute (that's barely a food!). There are lots of healthier indulgences on the market now, and, of course, there are those wonderful treats you can make at home, where you can control what goes into them. Occasionally, though, things will be out of your control. It's okay; you don't have to deny yourself the joy of eating a piece of birthday cake with family when you're eating well the rest of the time.

DEFENSIVE DINING: WHAT YOU *DON'T* WANT TO SEE ON THE INGREDIENTS LIST

Whenever I buy packaged foods, my personal philosophy is to look for ones that have relatively few ingredients and ingredients that I can pronounce. That just makes it easier to stay out of trouble—you'd have to be a chemist to decipher which of the hundreds of additives used in foods are safe but just sound bad and which genuinely *are* bad. For edification, I turn to the Center for Science in the Public Interest (CSPI), a watchdog group that's been advocating for food safety and nutrition since 1971. To see their list of food additives to avoid or use caution with, go to cspinet.org/reports/chemcuisine.htm#dyes.

BUY ORGANIC

Let's define organic food right off the bat. According to USDA rules, to carry the USDA Organic label, food must be produced without the use of toxic pesticides and fertilizers, antibiotics, synthetic hormones, genetic engineering, sewage sludge (yes! that's a conventional farming input), or irradiation. No doubt when you read all those words, you're thinking something like *Of course I don't want any of that in my food*. Yet when you see a gleaming tomato or shiny apple in the market, it's hard to imagine that those beautiful edibles have been touched by anything toxic. They seem perfectly fine. Conventionally grown food, though, is not always fine, even if we don't see evidence of it as we walk through the produce aisles. In fact, sometimes conventionally grown food looks particularly robust and healthy only because extreme measures have been taken to keep it free from pests or to grow varieties that stand up to shipping because all the good stuff (like flavor and nutrients) has been bred right out of them. Looks can be deceiving.

I started choosing organic food when I was in the thick of battling my autoimmune diseases. At that point, I had tried all different kinds of ways to eat, including a macrobiotic diet, hoping they'd work some kind of magic on me. Nothing did. However, once I made the switch to primarily organic foods, I felt significantly better, and my symptoms began to dissipate. Throwing chia into the mix put me over the top, and I've been symptom free ever since.

I can't tell you exactly why eating organically changed everything for me, but I sense that I am extremely sensitive to the chemicals used in conventional farming. Not everyone seems to be as vulnerable, yet I still believe in organic for all. I'll give you three good reasons why.

1. More Nutrients for Your Body—Organic growing methods utilize composted soil, which releases nitrogen slowly, allowing plants to grow at a normal rate with their nutrients in balance. To the contrary, vegetables grown with conventional fertilizers grow very rapidly and allocate less energy to developing nutrients. I don't want to overstate this, because the research looking at whether organic produce has more nutrients than conventionally grown produce is mixed. Stanford researchers, for instance, found no appreciable difference in the amounts of vitamins A, C, and E in organic and conventional produce when they reviewed a group of studies. But then you have studies like the 2003 one from the University of California at Davis (UC Davis), which found that at least two organic crops, corn and berries, had 58 percent more antioxidants than the same crops grown with chemicals. Other UC Davis research showed that organic spinach had higher levels of vitamin C and flavonoids and lower levels of detrimental nitrates than spinach grown conventionally. So while there is no conclusive study proving that all organic produce is better for you than any nonorganic versions, the potential for a difference is undeniable.

2. Fewer Chemicals for Your Body—Without sounding alarmist, I think it's important to note that pesticides have been linked to cancer and hormone disruption as well as injury to the brain and nervous system. More than 60 percent of Americans tested positive for seven or more pesticides and pesticide metabolites in a 2009 Centers for Disease Control study. Conventionally produced animals are often overtreated with antibiotics, which may be contributing to the development of bacteria that are resistant to treatment. In fact, the FDA is set to phase out the use of antibiotics in livestock, because once these superbugs get loose, antibiotics won't work when we really need them. What's more, when manure from antibiotic-treated animals is used on crops, the drugs can wind up in vegetables like corn, lettuce, and potatoes. Thus, consuming organic animal products can also lower your exposure to potentially harmful elements in food.

3. A Cleaner Environment—By supporting businesses that use organic farming methods, you can help reduce the amount of chemicals that gets into the environment, disrupting the ecosystem as well as damaging human lives. Chemical inputs from farming don't just end up in our food supply; they also end up in lakes and streams, forests and grasslands—essentially, everywhere—and they wreak all kinds of havoc, adding carbon dioxide to the air and killing and causing odd physiological changes in fish and animals, to say nothing of the effects on farmworkers and people who live near farms. In 2004, as part of an Agricultural Health Study, a large investigation in Iowa and North Carolina, researchers from the University of North Carolina, Chapel Hill, reported that children of farmworkers were at an increased risk for cancer. Some research also suggests that exposure to synthetic pesticides and fertilizers put those in the line of fire at greater risk for diseases like cancer and Parkinson's.

I'm happy to report that more and more people are seeing the light about organic food. When the Organic Trade Association did a survey in 2013, 81 percent of U.S. families reported purchasing organic food at least sometimes, and those who bought organic food bought more of it than they did the year before.

As much as I'm one of organic food's biggest cheerleaders, I'm also a realist. Organic food can be more expensive, it's not always readily available (although I am delighted that almost all mainstream grocery stores have an organic produce section now), and friends who invite you for dinner might not be as choosy as you. So don't make yourself crazy. Consider your budget and availability (see "When Organic Matters Most [and Least]," page 63). Remember that it's your total diet that's going to determine your health—not the one meal when you ate conventionally grown carrots. Pat yourself on the back for buying organic when you're able. And be the grateful and gracious guest I know you already are! I've had the experience of getting caught up in that "uh-oh" mentality, in which you establish some health-related policies for yourself and freak out a bit when you can't uphold your "doctrine." But consider all we eat in a day. Every ingredient in every meal doesn't have to be perfect. Think about the big picture: make eating healthy whole foods your number one priority, and eat organic whenever you can.

HOW CAN YOU BE SURE IT'S ORGANIC?

In most cases, you can tell if a food is organic by its label. It will either have the USDA Organic seal or that of another certifying agency. Organic produce generally has stickers with a five-digit PLU code that begins with a "9" (whereas nonorganic codes begin with a "4"). When there's no label or sticker, you'll have to rely on your seller, be it the owners of your grocery store or the group that runs your local farmers' market, to ensure that what they're selling is genuine. When a product has several ingredients and is labeled 100% Organic and USDA Organic, every ingredient must be organic. If not all the ingredients are organic, but 95 percent of them are, the product can still carry the USDA Organic seal. (If a product has 70 percent organic ingredients, manufacturers can label the individual ingredients organic if they choose but can't call the whole product USDA Organic.)

The labeling system is a great guide for selecting food, but it's not the only one. Becoming certified can be a challenging process for farmers; they have to spend considerable time and money to get certification. Many small farmers opt not to get certified for those reasons, though they still practice organic or sustainable (a less rigorous, but still environmentally sound method) farming. When you visit farmers' markets and roadside stands and don't see signs that promise organic, take the time to ask. Is it organic? Do you spray pesticides? Do you use synthetic fertilizers or herbicides? You'll find you may have many more options than you thought. And it is a great opportunity to build relationships with your local growers.

SEEDS OF KNOWLEDGE

. . . .

WHEN ORGANIC MATTERS MOST (AND LEAST)

Whether you're minding your wallet or just making a decision about whether to buy a particular nonorganic fruit or vegetable at all, it's helpful to know which items in the produce department tend to have the most pesticide residue. The Environmental Working Group (EWG) has been monitoring crops and continually updating which have the most and least amounts of residue. Based on that data, they recommend choosing organic whenever possible for these fruits and vegetables: apples, celery, cherry tomatoes, cucumbers, grapes, hot peppers, imported nectarines, peaches, potatoes, spinach, strawberries, sweet bell peppers, kale and collard greens, and summer squash. The organization found the cleanest produce (and the safest to buy conventionally grown) was asparagus, avocados, cabbage, cantaloupe, sweet corn, eggplant, grapefruit, kiwi, mangos, mushrooms, onions, papaya, pineapple, frozen sweet peas, and sweet potatoes. I would add some caveats to that list. Be aware that eggplant, papaya, and corn are often GMO, so even if they are low in pesticide residue, you may still want to go with organic. To learn more about avoiding pesticides while shopping, go to the EWG website, ewg.org/foodnews/summary.php.

GO NON-GMO

Remember how a few pages back I said that organic food sales are on the rise? Well, sales of food carrying non-GMO labels are rising even faster. To my mind, that's great news because it means that more people are getting the word that GMOs—short for genetically modified organisms—pose a danger to our health and to the health of agriculture in this country.

GMOs are genetically engineered plants or animals that have been created by inserting the DNA of one species into another, producing an organism that cannot occur in nature or be generated through traditional crossbreeding techniques. One of the primary reasons behind genetically engineering crops is to create plants that are resistant to herbicides—thereby allowing farmers to pour on chemicals that decimate weeds while leaving their crops unscathed. But that doesn't mean that GMO crops aren't contaminated; GMOs have the potential to contain even more chemical residue than usual.

And that's just one of the problems. GMOs often introduce new elements into foods that aren't there naturally, which can cause allergies and have potentially damaging side effects. Because they can spread from field to field, GMOs can also contaminate other crops— it's like the genie getting out of the bottle (with none of the fun shenanigans). Industry seems to be charging ahead even though there's not enough research to show that genetically modified foods are safe. What's more, there's very little oversight: the FDA doesn't require safety studies for GMO foods or labeling to indicate what products contain GMO ingredients.

There are a few ways to avoid GMOs. First, know where they live. The most common GMO crops are alfalfa, canola, corn, cotton, papaya, soy, sugar beets, zucchini, and yellow summer squash. Second, check labels. While there are no labeling requirements, some manufacturers want it known that their foods are GMO-free. You'll

SEEDS OF WISDOM

If you really want to make a friend, go to someone's house and eat with him. . . .The people who give you their food give you their heart.

—CESAR CHAVEZ, *leader of the farmworker rights movement*

know you're in the clear if you see a seal that says Non-GMO Project Verified or GMO Free Certified on packaged food. Third, keep up with organic eating. If they want to call their food organic, manufacturers' and growers' products can't be genetically modified. But take care: all certified organic products are non-GMO, but not all non-GMO certified products are organic.

ADVOCATE FOR YOUR RIGHT TO KNOW ABOUT GMO

People concerned about genetically modified foods are starting to get active, demanding that our government pass laws that mandate labeling on GMOs. One initiative on the California ballot failed, but we're not giving up! By being a supporter of GMO labeling, you can encourage the United States to join with sixty-four countries throughout the world, from Great Britain to Japan and Australia, that already ensure that genetically engineered foods are properly marked. Check out justlabelit.org and nongmoproject.org for more information.

GET THE FRESHEST POSSIBLE FOOD

Among chia's outstanding qualities is the fact that it's so shelf stable. You don't have to worry about its going bad quickly or losing key nutrients before you get around to using it. Not so with many of the other foods we depend on for vitality. Most fruits and vegetables begin losing vitamins and phytochemicals as soon as they're picked, so time is of the essence—you want to get them as fresh from the farmer's field as possible. Even foods that seem to hold up in the crisper are surreptitiously letting go of their beneficial compounds each hour they're off the vine. I was shocked to learn that broccoli loses up to 75 percent of its flavonoids and 50 percent of its vitamin C ten days after being picked and that it can take a week or more for it to travel from the field where it was picked to your friendly neighborhood supermarket.

To my mind, that's just one more reason to be deliberate about where you get your food. Here are three optimal options.

1. Farmers' Markets—I can give you a hundred and one reasons to shop at your local farmers' market, but in the interest of space, I'll narrow it down to five: (1) You'll likely find a good assortment of organic or no-spray vendors at the farmers' market. Plus you have the advantage of being able to meet your food suppliers (or those who work for them). Ask all the questions you want! (2) You'll be supporting local agriculture. Prefer to have farms near your community rather than subdivisions? I thought so. Keep those farmers in business! (3) You can eat seasonally. This will save you from wasting your money on peaches in winter only to find that these mealy flown-in-from-the-tropics stone fruits are not worth the money (think of the carbon footprint, too). (4) The food tastes better. Big industrial farms either pick their produce before it's ripe or breed it for sturdiness—they want foods that can stand up to being shipped around the country. Either way, flavor suffers. Small farmers, on the other hand, have the luxury of allowing their food to ripen on the vine since they sell direct to customers. (5) Talk about a sensual experience. The heady smell of herbs, the gorgeous stacks of greens, the glee at finding your favorite fruit has just come into season—a trip to the farmers' market makes you feel glad to be alive!

2. Community-Supported Agriculture (CSA)—This is a great way to buy seasonal local food right from the farmer who raised it. There are different CSA models, but typically, CSAs deliver a box of fresh food—fruits and vegetables, generally, but also sometimes eggs, cheese, poultry, or meat—to your door (or to a pickup location) for a regular fee. It's an ongoing subscription that allows you to invest in a farm. What I love about CSAs is the way they allow you to be a part of agriculture even if you live in a high-rise apartment. It's also fun to open the box every week and discover new produce that you might not have bought yourself—or even haven't seen before. You can usually opt out of foods you don't like ("Not a fan of bell peppers, bring me double carrots"), but belonging to a CSA also helps you expand your gastronomic horizons. You might not have selected artichokes at the market yourself, but when they turn up on your doorstep, you have the perfect opportunity to figure out how to use them. Check out localharvest.org/csa to find a CSA near you.

3. Grow Your Own—I live on an avocado farm, so I can vouch for the fact that there's nothing quite like eating something you've grown yourself. Friends, too, tell me they get a burst of childlike excitement when they bite into plants they started from seeds just a few weeks before. Gardening isn't for everyone, but if you have the space to grow your own—even a few pots you can devote to herbs or greens—you'll be getting the freshest food possible. My own travels tell me that more and more people are taking the plunge, cultivating edibles wherever they can. As I walk or drive down city and suburban streets these days I see Swiss chard and zucchini growing where there once were green lawns and rosebushes. All I can think about when I see those sprouting veggies is *Yum!* Somebody is in for a treat.

Chia can really rock your world when you work it into a diet of foods that are beautiful, nutritious, and delicious. No matter how little time you have to prepare your own meals, give yourself the gift of food that delights all your senses and is filled with nourishing nutrients. That will allow you to feel more alive, stay healthy, and noticeably improve your zest for life.

4

• • • • • •

THE 30-DAY *CHIA VITALITY* MEAL PLAN AND CLEANSE

I am now about to introduce you to a meal plan that will increase your vitality for sure! This 30-day plan is not about deprivation, consuming healthied-up facsimiles of real food, or—even though I'm the founder of a chia food and beverage company—living on chia drinks and smoothies. It's a plan that lets you bite into a fresh bounty of fruits and vegetables, whole grains, nuts, legumes, fish, poultry, and, of course, lots and lots of chia, all whipped up into modern, flavorful dishes. Note, too, that the foods in this meal plan weren't just chosen as a vehicle for chia; they, too, have healthful qualities that ramp up the entire nutritional value of each meal. Sometimes I see chia referred to as a supplement. That's not how I think of it at all. Chia is a *food*, and that's all the more evident when you see how beautifully it works with all the other delicious whole foods in this 30-day plan.

Another, optional, part of this plan is the *Chia Vitality* 3-day cleanse. My idea of a healthful cleanse is one that provides concentrated nutrients during a brief time span and doesn't leave you feeling ravenous and depleted. In fact, it should be energizing! Some people, it must be said, do feel energized by living on a very pared-down diet for a few days, but I'm not one of them. I think you'll find that my 3-day cleanse gives you a sense of renewal—and is a great way to kick off the 30-day meal plan that follows it—without testing your willpower.

Here's all you need to know to get started on the plan and, if you like, the cleanse.

THE 30-DAY *CHIA VITALITY* MEAL PLAN

OVERVIEW

I'm not a calorie counter, but I know that many people like to know how many calories they're getting at each meal. This information can also be very helpful in determining what portion sizes are right for your body, particularly if you're trying to lose weight. The approximate calorie counts in the 30-day *Chia Vitality* meal plan are as follows:

Breakfast (400 calories)
Lunch (550 calories)
Dinner (550 calories)
Snacks (200 calories each)*
Bonus snacks: Enjoy up to 2 cups a day of raw veggies, such as carrots, celery, cucumber, red and green bell peppers, and tomatoes. Go organic when possible.

---

*Women: Choose 0 snacks per day for weight loss, 1 snack per day for weight maintenance.

Men: Choose 1 snack per day for weight loss; 2 snacks per day for weight maintenance.

If highly active, add 1 extra (200-calorie) snack of choice per day. When possible, plan snacks for times you're most active.

**CALORIES FOR WEIGHT MAINTENANCE AND
WEIGHT LOSS**

The calorie levels below are to be used as general guidance when following the 30-day meal plan. Many variables determine calorie needs, including how much you weigh, your muscle-to-fat ratio, and your activity level. I measure in at barely five feet, so a calorie count that works for a woman who's five feet ten isn't going to work for me. Consider your dimensions and what you know about your personal ability to burn calories (some people just have a speedy metabolism, others a sluggish one), and listen to your body; all these factors will help determine your calorie needs. If you need more help, check in with a professional (your doctor, for instance, or a registered dietitian/nutritionist), who can ensure that your specific nutritional needs are met.

> Women: Weight loss = 1,500 calories; maintenance = 1,700 calories; maintenance/lightly active = 1,900 calories; moderately/highly active = 2,100 calories
> Men: Weight loss = 1,700 calories; maintenance = 1,900 calories; maintenance/lightly active = 2,100 calories; moderately/highly active = 2,300 calories

To determine your activity level, go by these guidelines:
- *Lightly active* means you do only physical activity associated with typical day-to-day life.
- *Moderately active* means you engage in physical activity equivalent to walking about 1.5 to 3 miles per day at 3 to 4 miles per hour in addition to the light physical activity associated with typical day-to-day life.
- *Highly active* means you engage in physical activity equivalent to walking more than 3 miles per day at 3 to 4 miles per hour in addition to the light physical activity associated with typical day-to-day life.

SERVING SIZES
The easy-prep dishes in this meal plan are designed to serve one. Most of the recipes, however, serve more than one, so you have the option to feed family and friends—why not spread some of that *Chia Vitality* love around! You can also, of course, refrigerate or freeze the leftovers for later. Most recipes are used a couple of times in the 30 days, thus saving you time in the kitchen.

CHOICES
One of the goals of this meal plan is to help you to shop easily and to avoid food waste. For instance, if one day calls for half a grapefruit or

a few slices of avocado, you'll be able to use the rest soon after. The plan also has a balance of nutrients: about 20 percent of the calories come from protein, 48 percent from carbohydrate, and 32 percent from fat. It thus falls perfectly in line with current national nutritional guidelines of 10 to 35 percent protein, 45 to 65 percent carbohydrate, and 20 to 35 percent fat. It also follows the principles of a Mediterranean diet, being low in saturated fat and having 0 grams of trans fat. What's more, it's rich in dietary fiber, so be sure to drink plenty of water throughout the day (which is always a good idea anyway).

I think you'll get the best results if you stick to the plan as closely as possible; however, meals within this plan can be mixed and matched to meet your specific eating style. Breakfasts can be swapped with other breakfasts; snacks switched with other snacks; and lunches or dinners exchanged with other lunches or dinners. In particular, if you are a vegetarian, there are several vegetarian meals that can be swapped for nonvegetarian dishes. If you're planning to dine out for lunch or dinner, try to choose approximately 4 ounces of lean poultry, fish, or tofu plus 1 cup of whole grains (or 2 slices of whole grain, gluten-free, or sprouted-grain bread) plus 1 to 2 cups of cooked veggies plus a little healthy fat, such as olive oil. You can use the Day 1 dinner as a model.

Naturally, the goal behind this plan is to give you 30 blissful, vitality-boosting days. But I also wanted to demonstrate how easy it is to incorporate chia into your diet. I want to make it so easy for you to eat chia that you'll start adding it to all the recipes in your usual repertoire. Believe me, I've seen it happen before. One minute, someone doesn't know what chia is; the next minute, the tiny seeds start showing up in all their favorite foods. Now that's the kind of conversion I can get behind!

This plan was also designed to meet the needs of as many types of eaters as possible as well as to reflect real-life eating. Surveying other types of meal plans, I noticed that the number of ingredients they use can be widely varied and that meals rarely repeat. Such an approach can certainly keep your meals interesting, but that's not how I and most of the people I know eat. I think this plan achieves a happy medium, avoiding meal and snack tedium, but respecting time, effort, and budget. You'll see that all the recipes, which begin on page 158, are easy to make. So are the easy-prep recipes, which are the simple instructions on how to assemble and maybe lightly cook a dish that you'll see worked into the meal plan grid (see page 82).

NO GLUTEN

There's probably no sector of the food market growing faster than gluten-free products. Sales of gluten-free foods were $4.2 billion in 2012, nearly *triple* what they were in 2008. Gluten-free products have become so abundant that the USDA even had to step in to set a standard to protect consumers from manufacturers trying to ride the lucrative gluten-free train. (The new standard for being considered gluten free is no more than 20 parts gluten per million [ppm], but some gluten-free foods may have less. Mamma Chia drinks and Chia Squeezes, for instance, test at 3 ppm.)

So many people are discovering that they're sensitive to gluten, and some are even finding that they have celiac disease, an autoimmune disorder and serious form of gluten intolerance, that I thought it would be helpful to make this plan gluten free. (Chia, as I've mentioned, is naturally gluten free.) I'm not overly sensitive to gluten, but I do try to eat only minimal amounts of wheat, which is one of the most common sources of gluten. The issue I have with wheat stems from what I see as one of the predominant sins of big agriculture. In order to make wheat heartier to withstand extreme weather conditions and yield bigger crops, it's been hybridized to death, stripping away some of its nutritional value and making it harder to digest and perhaps even harmful (inflammation may be one side effect). It also has more gluten now than the wheat eaten by generations before us, and some experts think the advent of this high-gluten wheat is why gluten sensitivities and celiac disease are coming to the forefront.

If gluten presents no problem for you, feel free to substitute regular breads, pastas, and crackers in recipes that call for gluten-free ones.

THE SPROUTED ALTERNATIVE

Even if gluten hasn't presented a noticeable problem for you, you may want to reduce your intake to see if it makes a difference in how you feel. A good place to start is with sprouted-grain products, which you'll see listed in the meal plan as an alternative to some gluten-free baked goods. Sprouted grains still contain gluten (they may be wheat or other gluten-containing grains, such as rye, barley, and contaminated oats), but there's some indication that, because sprouting starts the breakdown of gluten, they may be easier to digest.

There are several products with sprouted grains on the market, and you may be able to find local bakers who use them. I personally like the Northern California company Alvarado Street Bakery, but Food for Life's nationally distributed Ezekiel brand sprouted-grain breads are more readily available and tasty, too.

NO RED MEAT

If I thought that everyone had access to meats from grass-fed animals that have been raised humanely and without antibiotics, I might have included red meat in this diet. I am fortunate enough to live in an area where you can find beef and other meat produced in a conscientious manner, and I'm happy to say that the distribution of these products is becoming wider. But as it is, they're still somewhat hard to find and can be price prohibitive for some budgets.

That's one reason there's no red meat on the *Chia Vitality* 30-day meal plan. The other reason is that I wanted to make these 30 days a time when you might contemplate eating less meat or no red meat at all (I eat meat myself, but only occasionally). Thirty days with no meat may help you expand your culinary horizons and get you in the habit of eating in a healthier fashion. As you have probably already heard, regular meat eating increases the risk of cancer, heart disease, and diabetes. Less well known is that, according to Worldwatch Institute, an independent research organization, raising animals for food contributes 18 percent of greenhouse gases; some estimates even say it's closer to 51 percent—in my book, all good reasons to eat less meat.

SEEDS OF KNOWLEDGE

SELECT SEAFOOD WISELY

Fish, especially fatty fish like albacore tuna, salmon, and Alaskan halibut, are the richest sources of omega-3s. But the best? Not always. You might remember that in chapter 2, I mentioned that one of the reasons researchers were compelled to look at how well the body uses vegetarian omega-3s was because of dwindling and contaminated supplies of seafood. They were right to be concerned: The oceans are severely overfished, being depleted at rates that may make it hard for fish populations to come back. Many fish—particularly some forms of tuna, swordfish, orange roughy, mackerel, and shark—are also high in mercury: not a side dish you want with your omega-3s! We love our wild fish, but at what cost? And while farmed fish are helping to make up for some of the loss, some fish farming is associated with pollution and with damaging natural habitats. Sometimes farmed fish even escape and interbreed with local species, changing the gene pool of the natives and possibly affecting the natural ecology. Your best bet when choosing farmed fish is to buy varieties farmed in the United States.

This is unappetizing stuff, but if you're careful, you can safely navigate the waters. I am a huge fan of the Monterey Bay Aquarium's Seafood Watch. This program gives health-conscious eaters like us the most updated information on the best seafood choices as it continually monitors the science on ocean ecosystems. The program also makes it easy for shoppers by providing a Seafood

Watch app for some phones and printed pocket guides you can carry with you to stores and restaurants. I love the pocket guide! Check out the Seafood Watch website at http://www.monterey bayaquarium.org/cr/cr_seafoodwatch.

The fish called for in the 30-day meal plan was chosen according to Seafood Watch guidelines. For instance, I recommend wild salmon instead of farmed because much of salmon farmed these days has high levels of polychlorinated biphenyls (PCBs) and requires copious amounts of wild fish to produce (U.S.-farmed coho salmon is an exception). I also recommend that when you use canned tuna you look for varieties that have been troll or pole-and-line caught. Other methods of fishing can scoop up endangered species like sea turtles, sharks, and seabirds. The Soft Fish Tacos (page 175) call for barramundi or tilapia, two fish that are typically farmed. As noted above, look for U.S.-farmed varieties.

Buying fish that's been caught or produced in an eco-friendly way can cause a little sticker shock—it's definitely more expensive. But you won't be eating a lot of it (and you'll be saving money by not eating meat on this plan!), so think of it as a worthwhile expense. Think, too, about taking the time to find the origins of the fish you're buying. I know it's so much easier to just grab a package from the seafood section or to ask the counter person to wrap up your order and skedaddle out of the store. That extra minute of investigation, though, will be good for your health and the planet's health, too.

LOW SUGAR

Life will be sweeter, and you'll be healthier, if you keep your sugar intake at a moderate level. We hear a lot about how too much sugar isn't good for us, and research bears this out: High-sugar diets are associated with inflammation, high blood pressure, high cholesterol, and high triglycerides. High sugar intake may even make you a little dim-witted. Testing the theory on rats, UCLA researchers found that copious amounts of high-fructose corn syrup caused the animals to have diminished brain activity, including memory function. Interestingly, omega-3s minimized the damage in one group of rats. Just another reason to eat more chia! Processed foods are one of the biggest sources of sugar in the diet; however, just by virtue of being based primarily on whole foods, the *Chia Vitality* 30-day plan is automatically low in sugar. Of course, I want this plan to be a sweet experience for you, so I've taken care to find a balance of adding just enough sweetener (in most cases, less processed sweeteners such as maple syrup or agave nectar) to be yummy, but not so much that it's unhealthful.

OTHER OPTIONS

You'll see as you read through the meal plan and the cleanse (more on that below) that I don't always mention that the foods you choose should be organic. By now you know I'm a fierce proponent of organic foods, so consider it implied, but I leave it up to you. Do the best that you can. You'll also notice that occasionally I'll recommend a brand name. I really appreciate it when people give me brand-name tips, so I thought I'd pass on the favor. Consider these recommendations entirely optional, of course.

What follows are more specifics about both the 3-day cleanse and the 30-day plan. *Bon appétit!*

THE 3-DAY *CHIA VITALITY* CLEANSE

If you are looking for a kick start to help set you on the right track to healthful eating, you can try this (totally optional) 3-day 1,500-calorie cleanse before starting the *Chia Vitality* 30-day meal plan. It's a well-balanced, fully satisfying program with the stamina-enhancing benefits of chia. The cleanse calls for smoothie-like drinks in the morning and later in the afternoon but allows you to have full, nourishing meals for lunch and dinner. You don't need a special juicing machine to make the smoothies, just a regular kitchen blender, and because you'll repeat the menu each day, there is not a lot of shopping or work involved over the three days. The plan is flexible, too; you can dine out for dinner if you like and still follow the plan.

One final note: This plan is designed for nearly everyone to follow. However, for a vegan version, you can replace the regular yogurt with about ½ cup plain Greek-style cultured almond or coconut milk yogurt. For a weight loss version of this plan, skip the afternoon Chia Vitality Recharger P.M., or select the lower-calorie versions of both the A.M. and P.M. Chia Vitality Rechargers. If you're highly active, consider adding an evening snack—or another Chia Vitality Recharger P.M. As noted in the beginning of this book, before following any diet, check in with your doctor.

Breakfast
Chia Vitality Recharger A.M. (page 78)
15 whole raw almonds or raw walnuts

Morning Snack
½ cup plain fat-free Smári Icelandic yogurt or Greek yogurt sprinkled with 2 tablespoons fresh or thawed frozen blueberries and ½ teaspoon black chia seeds
OR 1 hard-boiled egg

Lunch
3 cups packed fresh baby spinach tossed with 2½ ounces roasted lean poultry or baked organic tofu cubes, 2 teaspoons extra-virgin olive oil, 1 tablespoon sliced raw almonds, 1½ teaspoons black chia seeds, lemon juice or apple cider vinegar to taste, and fresh herbs, such as mint or cilantro, to taste
1 ounce whole grain gluten-free or sprouted-grain roll or brown rice crackers

Afternoon Snack
Chia Vitality Recharger P.M. (page 79)

Dinner

4 ounces grilled or roasted lean poultry, fish, or organic tofu "steak," served with a lemon wedge

1 cup steamed quinoa or brown rice, pinch of sea salt, and fresh herbs, such as cilantro or dill, to taste

2 cups veggies of choice sautéed in 1 teaspoon extra-virgin olive oil

Nutritional information (per day): 1500 calories, 48 g total fat, 7 g saturated fat, 0 g trans fat, 155 mg cholesterol, 670 mg sodium, 183 g total carbohydrate, 38 g dietary fiber, 80 g sugars, 100 g protein.

Cleanse Recipes

CHIA VITALITY RECHARGER A.M. (morning)

Enjoying this nourishing smoothie-style cleanse first thing in the morning will give you a true energy boost without caffeine. It's loaded with health-promoting plant nutrients and has a significant amount of fiber. Use organic ingredients when possible.

Makes 2½ cups

1 medium mango, peeled, seeded, chopped, and frozen, or 1 cup frozen mango cubes

1 cup cucumber, peeled, seeded, and chopped

½ cup Chia Gel (page 157), chilled

½ cup 100% pure organic apple juice (not from concentrate)*

½ packed cup fresh baby spinach or kale leaves (about 1 handful)

2 tablespoons fresh mint leaves

2 tablespoons fresh flat-leaf parsley leaves

1 tablespoon fresh lemon juice or apple cider vinegar, or to taste

Pinch of cayenne pepper

In a blender, purée all the ingredients until very smooth. Drink immediately.

Per serving: 230 calories, 4 g total fat, 0.5 g saturated fat, 0 g trans fat, 0 mg cholesterol, 35 mg sodium, 49 g total carbohydrate, 8 g dietary fiber, 36 g sugars, 5 g protein.

*For a lower-calorie option and fewer sugar grams, replace the ½ cup apple juice with ½ cup cold filtered water, 2 packets organic stevia, and an extra 2 teaspoons fresh lemon juice. Per serving: 180 calories, 4 g total fat, 0.5 g saturated fat, 0 g trans fat, 0 mg cholesterol, 30 mg sodium, 38 g total carbohydrate, 8 g dietary fiber, 25 g sugars, 4 g protein.

· ·

CHIA VITALITY RECHARGER P.M. (afternoon)

This satisfying blueberry-ginger drink is ideal after a workout or after work when you might be feeling a little sluggish. It's loaded with antioxidants.

Makes 2 cups

> *1 cup blueberries, frozen, or 1 6-ounce package frozen blueberries*
> *½ cup 100% pure organic apple juice (not from concentrate)**
> *½ cup Chia Gel (page 157), chilled*
> *2 tablespoons fresh mint leaves*
> *2 teaspoons fresh lemon juice or apple cider vinegar, or to taste*
> *1 teaspoon freshly grated ginger*
> *Pinch of cayenne pepper*

In a blender, purée all the ingredients until very smooth and only tiny flecks of blueberry skin remain. Drink immediately.

Per serving: 210 calories, 3.5 g total fat, 0 g saturated fat, 0 mg cholesterol, 10 mg sodium, 44 g total carbohydrate, 8 g dietary fiber, 29 g sugars, 3 g protein.

*For a lower-calorie option and fewer sugar grams, replace the ½ cup apple juice with ½ cup cold filtered water, 2 packets organic stevia, and an extra 2 teaspoons fresh lemon juice. Per serving: 160 calories, 3.5g total fat, 0g saturated fat, 0mg cholesterol, 0mg sodium, 32g total carbohydrate, 8g dietary fiber, 17g sugars, 3g protein.

THE *CHIA VITALITY* KITCHEN

Rather than have you comb through all the recipes to see what basics you need to have on hand, I've assembled this list of the pantry, refrigerator, and freezer staples you'll need during the next 30 days. You'll notice that I sometimes specify organic when I think it's particularly important; but while, of course, it's always a matter of choice, ideally you'll stock up with mostly organic, non-GMO products.

Pantry Staples

- Chia seeds: black chia seeds, white chia seeds, and milled/ground chia seeds
- Spices: sea salt, pepper, cinnamon, hot pepper flakes, ground cumin, ground coriander, chili powder, ground or fresh nutmeg, cayenne pepper
- Oils: extra-virgin olive oil (preferably organic), unrefined coconut oil, sesame oil, cooking spray
- Vinegars: brown or regular rice, apple cider, balsamic, white balsamic (lemon juice can be substituted)
- Tamari soy sauce
- Worcestershire sauce
- Low-sodium broths: organic chicken, vegetable
- Pure extract: vanilla
- Sweeteners: local honey or organic agave nectar, organic brown sugar, maple syrup
- Flours: buckwheat, gluten-free all-purpose baking, garbanzo bean (chickpea)
- Onions: garlic, red and white onions
- Whole grains: short-grain brown rice, brown basmati rice, quinoa, whole grain gluten-free spaghetti
- Whole grain gluten-free cereal flakes
- Buckwheat soba noodles
- Gluten-free crackers (my favorites are Mary's Gone Crackers)

- Canned goods: crushed roasted organic tomatoes, vegetarian refried black beans, low-sodium organic Great Northern or cannellini or dried white beans, black or pinto beans
- Nuts and seeds (raw and unsalted unless noted): pecans, sliced almonds, whole almonds, roasted pumpkin seeds, walnuts, pine nuts, roasted salt-and-pepper or regular pistachios, roasted sunflower seeds
- Nut butters: creamy no-added-sugar peanut, almond
- Dried fruit: tart cherries or cranberries, raisins
- Tea: green tea

Fridge Staples

- Butter, vegan or regular
- Eggs, cage-free and organic
- Citrus: lemons, limes, and oranges (the latter for making fresh orange juice)
- Grainy Dijon mustard
- Mayonnaise, vegan or regular
- Ginger
- Serrano peppers
- Plain unsweetened almond milk or other plant-based milk
- Cheeses: Parmigiano-Reggiano or Pecorino Romano, Monterey Jack, soft goat, Neufchâtel (light cream cheese)
- Yogurt, plain fat-free Icelandic or Greek
- Salsa
- Bread: whole grain gluten-free or sprouted-grain English muffins, hamburger buns, hot dog buns, rolls*

*A NOTE ON BREAD
Some people like to buy bread fresh weekly (or even daily), others like to buy it ahead of time and store it in the freezer. If you opt to do the latter, this list tells you what to buy at the outset of this program. It also gives you the option of choosing gluten-free breads or sprouted grain. For sprouted-grain products I like Food for Life.

THE *CHIA VITALITY* 30-DAY PLAN

Most but not every meal here contains chia. Feel free to add a teaspoon or two as you go. One note about two of the ingredients in this plan. Several of the recipes and easy-prep ideas call for corn and corn products like corn tortillas. Corn is so delicious, but note that most of the corn on the market these days (about 88 percent) is GMO. Whenever possible, look for verified non-GMO varieties of corn and soy products (buying organic will guarantee they're non-GMO); that's a good way to keep corn and soy on your plate and still get food that's good for you.

V = Vegetarian

DAY 1	
Breakfast (400 calories)	**Avocado Toast and Ricotta (V)** 1 slice whole grain gluten-free or sprouted-grain toast, topped with ¼ mashed Hass avocado, squirt of lemon juice, 1 egg cooked "over easy" in a cooking spray–coated nonstick skillet; add fresh rosemary and sea salt to taste ½ cup part-skim ricotta cheese sprinkled with 1 teaspoon honey or agave nectar, ½ teaspoon chia seeds, and sea salt to taste
Lunch (550 calories)	**Thai Tofu Peanut Noodles, Orange, and Almonds (V)** 1 serving *Thai Tofu Peanut-Chia Noodles* (page 165) 1 large orange 10 raw almonds
Dinner (550 calories)	**Rotisserie Chicken, Rice, and Baby Spinach** 1 rotisserie chicken breast without skin or 4 ounces grilled chicken 1 cup cooked brown basmati rice with 1½ tablespoons toasted pine nuts (or sliced almonds) and fresh mint to taste 3 cups packed fresh baby spinach sautéed in 1 teaspoon extra-virgin olive oil, served with lemon wedge and sea salt to taste
Snacks (200 calories each)	**Chips and Salsa (V)** 14 blue or yellow corn tortilla chips with mixture of ¼ cup salsa and 1 tablespoon *Chia Gel* (page 157) **Brie and Grapes (V)** 1 1½-ounce wedge of Brie cheese with 18 red seedless grapes

DAY 2

Breakfast (400 calories)

Frittata, Raspberry-Topped Yogurt, and English Muffin (V)
1 serving *California Frittata* (page 160)
1 6-ounce container plain fat-free Smári Icelandic yogurt or Greek yogurt topped with ½ cup fresh or frozen thawed raspberries and sprinkled with ½ teaspoon chia seeds and, if desired, 1 teaspoon honey or agave nectar
½ whole grain gluten-free or sprouted-grain English muffin, toasted, with 1 teaspoon almond butter

Lunch (550 calories)

Turkey and Avocado Sandwich with Carrots and Hummus
1 whole grain gluten-free or sprouted-grain hamburger bun stuffed with ½ sliced Hass avocado, 3 ounces smoked turkey breast, 1 large slice of red onion, ½ cup baby arugula, and 2 teaspoons Dijon mustard
10 baby carrots with ¼ cup hummus or 1% low-sodium cottage cheese

Dinner (550 calories)

Caprese Spaghetti with Leafy Grape Salad (V)
1 cup cooked whole grain gluten-free spaghetti tossed with 2 ounces cubed part-skim mozzarella cheese, 1 diced medium tomato, 2 tablespoons chopped fresh basil, 1 minced garlic clove, 1½ teaspoons extra-virgin olive oil, and sea salt to taste
2 cups mixed baby salad greens with 8 red seedless grapes and 1½ teaspoons each: extra-virgin olive oil, balsamic vinegar, and chia seeds

Snacks (200 calories each)

Tart Cherries and Pistachios (V)
⅓ cup dried tart cherries with 15 roasted pistachios

Tropical Smoothie (V)
¾ cup fresh pineapple cubes blended into a smoothie with ½ cup fat-free vanilla frozen yogurt, ¼ cup fresh orange juice, and 2 teaspoons *Chia Gel* (page 157)

DAY 3

Breakfast (400 calories)

Strawberry-Topped Cereal and Banana (V)
1¼ cups whole grain gluten-free cereal flakes with 1 cup fat-free milk, ⅓ cup sliced fresh or frozen thawed strawberries, sprinkled with 2 teaspoons chia seeds
1 small banana

Lunch (550 calories)	**Middle Eastern Mezze Meal (V)** ½ cup hummus, 1 cup sliced cucumber, 10 small gluten-free whole grain crackers, such as Mary's Gone Crackers ¾ cup tabouli or vegetable-based salad (from deli)
Dinner (550 calories)	**Curry Turkey Burger, Quinoa, and Red Peppers** 1 serving *Indian-Spiced Turkey Burgers with Chia Curry Ketchup* (page 178) 1 cup cooked quinoa, prepared with 2 teaspoons chia seeds; stir in 1 tablespoon chopped fresh cilantro 1 large sliced red pepper (or 1 sliced zucchini) sautéed with 1 teaspoon unrefined virgin coconut oil
Snacks (200 calories each)	**Edamame with Sea Salt (V)** 1 cup cooked edamame in pods with sea salt to taste **Fruity Smoothie (V)** 1 serving *Chia Cherry Vanilla Smoothie* (page 191)

DAY 4

Breakfast (400 calories)	**Almond Butter and Banana Toastie (V)** 2 slices whole grain gluten-free or sprouted-grain bread filled with 1½ tablespoons almond butter, ½ teaspoon chia seeds, and ½ sliced small banana; toast in cooking spray–coated skillet or panini press ½ small banana
Lunch (550 calories)	**Tuna Salad Platter** 1 serving *Mediterranean Tuna Salad* (page 164) 20 small gluten-free whole grain crackers, such as Mary's Gone Crackers ½ cup hummus with 2 medium celery stalks
Dinner (550 calories)	**Chicken Pesto Pasta with Red Peppers** 1½ cups cooked whole grain gluten-free spaghetti tossed with 2 tablespoons each pesto sauce and *Chia Gel* (page 157), 3 ounces shredded rotisserie chicken breast meat, ½ thinly sliced fresh red pepper (or ½ cup gently steamed sliced zucchini), and ½ minced serrano pepper

Berries and Frozen Yogurt (V)
¾ cup fat-free vanilla frozen yogurt topped with ½ cup fresh or frozen thawed berries of choice and sprinkled with ½ teaspoon chia seeds

Cheesy Corn Tortilla with Guacamole (V)
1 6-inch soft corn tortilla with 2 tablespoons shredded Monterey Jack cheese, warmed; serve with one serving *Chia Guacamole* (page 189) or 3 tablespoons other guacamole on the side

Snacks (200 calories each)

DAY 5

Mexican Breakfast Scramble (V)
Scramble 1 egg, 2 tablespoons *Chia Gel* (page 157), and 12 grape tomatoes in a cooking spray–coated nonstick skillet and stir in 6 blue or yellow corn tortilla chips and 1 ounce (¼ cup) shredded Monterey Jack cheese; serve with 2 tablespoons salsa and 1 serving *Chia Guacamole* (page 189) or 3 tablespoons other guacamole on the side

Breakfast (400 calories)

Citrus Rice Salad with Chicken
1 serving *Orange-Chia Rice Salad with Fresh Mint* (page 169)
4 ounces boneless, skinless pregrilled chicken breast or 1 rotisserie chicken breast with skin, reheated in microwave if necessary
1 cup 1% low-sodium cottage cheese (or ½ cup part-skim ricotta cheese) with 1 teaspoon each roasted sunflower seeds and honey or agave nectar

Lunch (550 calories)

Asian Salmon on Spinach with Veggies
1 serving *Asian Pan-Seared Chia-Crusted Salmon with Spinach* (page 176)
1 cup frozen thawed non-GMO corn or finely diced butternut squash, sautéed with 1 teaspoon extra-virgin olive oil and 1 minced scallion, served with lime wedge
1 ounce whole grain gluten-free or sprouted-grain roll

Dinner (550 calories)

Chocolate Raisins (V)
¼ cup chocolate-covered raisins

Shrimp Cocktail and Mamma Chia
10 large cooked chilled shrimp with 1½ tablespoons cocktail sauce; serve with 1 (10-ounce) bottle Mamma Chia Vitality Beverage or 1 (5-ounce) glass wine

Snacks (200 calories each)

DAY 6

Breakfast (400 calories)

Orange Smoothie Breakfast (V)
1¼ cups low-fat vanilla yogurt blended into a smoothie with ⅔ cup each fresh orange juice and low-fat (1%) milk (or plant-based milk), 2 tablespoons *Chia Gel* (page 157), and about 3 large ice cubes

Lunch (550 calories)

Baja Bean Salad with Corn Tortilla (V)
2 cups mixed baby salad greens tossed with ¾ cup pinto or black beans, 1 medium chopped green pepper (or 1 cup sliced white button mushrooms), ⅔ cup each frozen, thawed non-GMO corn, 1 ounce (¼ cup) shredded or cubed Monterey Jack cheese, 3 tablespoons salsa mixed with 1 tablespoon *Chia Gel* (page 157) and 1 teaspoon extra-virgin olive oil, and lime juice and fresh cilantro to taste
2 6-inch soft corn tortillas

Dinner (550 calories)

Eggplant Parm with Basil Quinoa (V)
3 large, thick slices eggplant, spritzed with olive oil cooking spray and grilled or roasted; top with ½ cup warm marinara sauce and 1½ ounces part-skim mozzarella cheese; place under the broiler to melt
1 cup steamed quinoa mixed with 1 tablespoon each toasted pine nuts and chopped fresh basil; add sea salt to taste

Snacks (200 calories each)

Snack Mix (V)
⅓ cup snack mix (dried fruit, nuts, and seeds) OR 1 (3.5-ounce) Mamma Chia Organic Chia Squeeze Vitality Snack + 3 tablespoons snack mix

Apple Crisp (V)
1 serving *Chia Oat Apple Crisp* (page 192)

DAY 7

Breakfast (400 calories)

Granola-Berry Sundae (V)
1 serving *Chia Granola* (page 159) layered in a sundae or other glass with 1 (6-ounce) container plain fat-free Smári Icelandic yogurt or Greek yogurt and ½ cup fresh or frozen, thawed strawberries or raspberries

Lunch (550 calories)

Double Salad Lunch (V)
1 serving *Chia Caesar Kale Salad* (page 170)
¾ cup cannellini or other white beans tossed with 1 teaspoon each extra-virgin olive oil and balsamic vinegar (or lemon juice), and fresh herbs to taste
1 1-ounce whole grain gluten-free or sprouted-grain roll
1 cup red or green seedless grapes

Dinner (550 calories)	**Veggie Stir-Fry with Ginger Rice (V)** 1 cup each fresh broccoli florets and sliced cremini or white button mushrooms, and 4 ounces extra-firm tofu stir-fried in 2 teaspoons sesame oil and tossed with 2 tablespoons all-natural kung pao or stir-fry sauce 1 cup steamed brown rice or wild rice with 1 teaspoon grated ginger and 1 teaspoon chia seeds
Snacks (200 calories each)	**Crackers and Dip (V)** 1 serving *Chia Edamame Dip* (page 188) with 13 small whole grain gluten-free crackers, such as Mary's Gone Crackers **Apple Crisp (V)** 1 serving *Chia Oat Apple Crisp* (page 192)

DAY 8

Breakfast (400 calories)	**Blueberry Pancakes and Yogurt (V)** 1 serving *Blueberry Buckwheat Pancakes* (page 162) 1 6-ounce container plain fat-free Smári Icelandic yogurt or Greek yogurt drizzled with 1 tablespoon chopped walnuts or pistachios and, if desired, 1 teaspoon honey or agave nectar
Lunch (550 calories)	**Veggie Sandwich and White Bean Salad (V)** 2 slices whole grain gluten-free or sprouted-grain bread stuffed with ½ cup each sliced roasted red or green pepper (or sliced grilled zucchini) and thinly sliced cucumber, 2 thin slices red onion, ½ cup fresh baby arugula, 1½ ounces soft goat cheese, and 1 teaspoon each extra-virgin olive oil and balsamic vinegar ¾ cup cannellini or other white beans tossed with 1 teaspoon each extra-virgin olive oil, balsamic vinegar, and chia seeds; add fresh herbs to taste
Dinner (550 calories)	**Rotisserie Chicken, Rice, and Baby Spinach** 1 rotisserie chicken breast without skin or 4 ounces grilled chicken 1 cup steamed brown basmati rice with 1 tablespoon toasted pine nuts (or sliced almonds), 1 teaspoon chia seeds, and fresh mint to taste 3 cups packed fresh baby spinach sautéed in 1 teaspoon extra-virgin olive oil, served with lemon wedge and sea salt to taste
Snacks (200 calories each)	**Almonds (V)** 25 raw almonds **Crackers and Chia Edamame Dip (V)** 1 serving *Chia Edamame Dip* (page 188) with 13 small whole grain gluten-free crackers, such as Mary's Gone Crackers

DAY 9

Breakfast (400 calories)

Oatmeal and Turkey Bacon
1 serving *Steel-Cut "Superfood" Oatmeal* (page 158)
1 ounce nitrite-free turkey bacon, such as Applegate Organics
    Uncured Turkey Bacon
2 kiwi fruits

Lunch (550 calories)

Turkey Wrap and Arugula Salad
1 large whole grain gluten-free wrap or sprouted-grain tortilla
    stuffed with 2½ ounces smoked turkey breast, ⅛ cup sliced red
    onion, 1 cup baby arugula, and 1 tablespoon honey mustard
2 cups baby arugula salad with 12 red seedless grapes, 1 ounce
    crumbled soft goat cheese, 1 tablespoon sliced almonds,
    2 teaspoons extra-virgin olive oil, and apple cider vinegar to taste

Dinner (550 calories)

Salmon with Veggie Fried Rice
5 ounces pan-grilled wild salmon or other fish, spritzed with olive
    oil cooking spray, sea salt, and freshly ground black pepper to
    taste
1 serving *Thai Basil Veggie Fried Rice* (page 186)

Snacks (200 calories each)

Mango Chia Yogurt (V)
¾ cup low-fat vanilla yogurt topped with ½ cup cubed mango or
    banana and ½ teaspoon chia seeds

Pear with Cheese (V)
1 pear, cut into wedges, with 1 ounce blue cheese or aged goat
    cheese

DAY 10

Breakfast (400 calories)

Granola and Grapefruit (V)
1 serving *Chia Granola* (page 159) with ½ cup low-fat (1%) milk or
    plant-based milk
½ large pink grapefruit with 1 teaspoon honey or agave nectar

Lunch (550 calories)

Sushi and Fruit
12-piece brown rice California sushi (from market or restaurant)
    with tamari soy sauce, pickled ginger, and wasabi paste to taste
½ large pink grapefruit with 1 teaspoon honey or agave nectar or
    2 kiwi fruits

Dinner (550 calories)	**Roasted Turkey with Beet and Goat Cheese Salad** 1 serving *Beet and Goat Cheese Salad* (page 185) 5 ounces turkey tenderloin brushed with 1 tablespoon horseradish or Dijon mustard and roasted at 400°F until well done, about 25 minutes, then seasoned with sea salt to taste 1 large baked sweet potato, sprinkled with 1 ounce crumbled soft goat cheese, 1 teaspoon chia seeds, and fresh basil to taste
Snacks (200 calories each)	**Pineapple and Smoked Turkey Skewers** 1½ ounces cubed smoked turkey on skewers with 1½ cups pineapple cubes **Cookie Break (V)** 1 cookie *Chia White Chocolate Macadamia Cookies* (page 190)

DAY 11

Breakfast (400 calories)	**Breakfast Crostini (V)** 1 whole grain gluten-free or sprouted-grain English muffin, split and toasted, each muffin half topped with ¼ cup part-skim ricotta cheese, ½ peeled and diced kiwi fruit, ¾ teaspoon honey or agave nectar, ¼ teaspoon chia seeds, and sea salt to taste
Lunch (550 calories)	**Chicken Salad with Grapes** 1 serving *Green Tea Chicken and Grape Salad* (page 168) 20 small gluten-free crackers, such as Mary's Gone Crackers 1 cup red or green seedless grapes
Dinner (550 calories)	**Eggplant Mozzarella with Basil Quinoa (V)** 3 large thick slices eggplant, spritzed with olive oil cooking spray, and grilled or roasted; top with ½ cup warm marinara sauce and 1½ ounces part-skim mozzarella cheese; place under the broiler to melt 1 cup steamed quinoa mixed with 1 tablespoon each toasted pine nuts and chopped fresh basil; add sea salt to taste
Snacks (200 calories each)	**Chocolate Pudding (V)** 1 serving *Chia Chocolate Pudding* (page 193), served with 3 large fresh strawberries if desired **Apple and Pistachios (V)** 1 small apple and 35 roasted or salt-and-pepper pistachios

DAY 12

Breakfast (400 calories)

Egg Muffin Sandwich (V)
1 egg "fried" in a cooking spray–coated nonstick skillet and served in a toasted whole grain gluten-free or sprouted-grain hamburger bun or English muffin with a 1-ounce slice of part-skim mozzarella cheese, 1 large slice of tomato, and ½ cup fresh baby arugula tossed with ½ teaspoon lemon juice
¾ cup cubed mango or other fruit

Lunch (550 calories)

Basmati Salad with Swiss-Turkey Rolls
1 serving *Dill Roasted Carrot and Basmati Salad* (page 172)
2 1-ounce slices deli roasted or smoked turkey, each rolled up with a ¾-ounce slice of Swiss cheese and ½ teaspoon Dijon mustard; secure each with a toothpick
1 small apple

Dinner (550 calories)

Chili Bowl with Salad
1 serving *Chicken Chia Chili* (page 181)
3 cups mixed baby salad greens lightly dressed with 2 teaspoons each extra-virgin olive oil and lime juice and ½ teaspoon chia seeds
2 6-inch soft corn tortillas
¾ cup cubed mango or other fruit

Snacks (200 calories each)

Almonds (V)
25 raw almonds

Dark Chocolate (V)
1¼-ounce portion dark chocolate bar (at least 60% cacao) or 4 Dagoba Organic New Moon Bittersweet Dark Chocolate squares

DAY 13

Breakfast (400 calories)

Bagel with Scallion Cream Cheese (V)
1 4-ounce toasted whole grain gluten-free or sprouted-grain bagel with 2 tablespoons Neufchâtel (light cream cheese) sprinkled with 1 minced scallion

Lunch (550 calories)

Tropical Quinoa and Kale with Soup (V)
1 serving *Tropical Quinoa and Kale* (page 166)
1½ cups low-sodium black bean or other soup (about 200 calories)
20 grape tomatoes, halved, and tossed with 1 teaspoon extra-virgin olive oil and sea salt to taste

Dinner (550 calories)

Asian Salmon on Spinach with Veggies
1 serving *Asian Pan-Seared Chia-Crusted Salmon with Spinach* (page 176)
1 cup frozen, thawed non-GMO corn or finely diced butternut squash, sautéed with 1 teaspoon extra-virgin olive oil and 1 minced scallion; serve with a lime wedge
1 1-ounce whole grain gluten-free or sprouted-grain roll

Snacks (200 calories each)

Fruity Smoothie (V)
1 serving *Chia Cherry Vanilla Smoothie* (page 191)

Berries and Frozen Yogurt (V)
¾ cup fat-free vanilla frozen yogurt topped with ½ cup fresh or frozen, thawed berries of choice and sprinkled with ½ teaspoon chia seeds

DAY 14

Breakfast (400 calories)

Yogurt with Strawberry Jam and Almonds (V)
1 cup plain fat-free Smári Icelandic yogurt or Greek yogurt topped with 1 serving *Fresh Strawberry–Chia Seed Jam* (page 161)
20 raw almonds
1 small banana

Lunch (550 calories)

Bagel Deli Melt and Cup of Soup
½ (2-ounce portion) whole grain gluten-free or sprouted-grain bagel, topped with 1 teaspoon Dijon mustard, 2 ounces lean ham or smoked turkey, and a 1-ounce slice of Swiss cheese; heat in the microwave until the cheese melts
1 cup reduced-sodium split pea soup (about 180 calories)
15 baby carrots

Dinner (550 calories)

Chicken Chia Chili Spaghetti
1 serving *Chicken Chia Chili* (page 181) (if possible, use leftovers from Day 12) tossed with 1¾ cups cooked whole grain gluten-free spaghetti

Snacks (200 calories each)

Apple with Almond Butter (V)
1 small apple cut into wedges with 4 teaspoons almond butter

Deviled Eggs (V)
1 hard-boiled egg, halved, yolk mixed with 2 teaspoons vegan mayonnaise and a pinch of cayenne pepper
15 baby carrots

DAY 15

Breakfast (400 calories)

Cinnamon Toast, Grapefruit, and Vanilla Milk (V)
1 slice whole grain gluten-free or sprouted-grain toast spread with
    1 teaspoon butter or vegan butter and sprinkled with ½ teaspoon
    honey or agave nectar and a pinch of cinnamon
½ large pink grapefruit with 1 teaspoon honey or agave nectar
1 cup almond or other plant-based vanilla milk
15 raw almonds

Lunch (550 calories)

Pear and Goat Cheese Salad with Chicken
1 serving *Mesclun Salad with Pear, Walnuts, and Goat Cheese*
    (page 173)
2 pregrilled boneless, skinless chicken thighs, warm or chilled
    (about 4 ounces each)

Dinner (550 calories)

Sausage and "Fries"
1 3-ounce link gluten-free poultry sausage, such as Applegate
    Organics Chicken & Apple Sausage, served on a whole grain
    gluten-free or sprouted-grain frankfurter bun with 2 teaspoons
    each ketchup, Dijon mustard, and minced red onion
1 serving *Chia Sweet Potato "Fries"* (page 179)
1 cup steamed baby spinach or zucchini, lemon wedge, and sea
    salt to taste
1 cup almond or other plant-based vanilla milk

Snacks (200 calories each)

Snack Mix (V)
⅓ cup snack mix (dried fruit, nuts, and seeds) OR 1 (3.5-
    ounce) Mamma Chia Organic Chia Squeeze Vitality Snack +
    3 tablespoons snack mix

Frozen Yogurt Sundae (V)
¾ cups fat-free mint or vanilla frozen yogurt or plant-based frozen
    dessert drizzled with mixture of 2 teaspoons each *Chia Gel* (page
    157) and organic chocolate syrup

DAY 16

Breakfast (400 calories)

Avocado Toast and Ricotta (V)
1 slice whole grain or sprouted-grain gluten-free toast, topped with
    ¼ mashed Hass avocado, squirt of lemon juice, 1 egg cooked
    "over easy" in a cooking spray–coated nonstick skillet; add fresh
    rosemary and sea salt to taste
½ cup part-skim ricotta cheese sprinkled with 1 teaspoon honey or
    agave nectar, ½ teaspoon chia seeds, and sea salt to taste

Lunch
(550 calories)

Middle Eastern Mezze Meal (V)
½ cup hummus, 1 cup sliced cucumber, 10 small gluten-free whole grain crackers, such as Mary's Gone Crackers
¾ cup tabouli or vegetable-based salad (from deli)

Dinner
(550 calories)

Fish Tacos and Guacamole
1 serving *Soft Fish Tacos with Chia Pico de Gallo* (page 175)
1 serving *Chia Guacamole* (page 189) or 3 tablespoons other guacamole
½ cup organic vegetarian refried beans
1 cup mango cubes or other fruit

Snacks
(200 calories each)

Tart Cherries and Pistachios (V)
⅓ cup dried tart cherries with 15 roasted pistachios

Tropical Smoothie (V)
¾ cup fresh pineapple cubes blended into a smoothie with ½ cup fat-free vanilla frozen yogurt, ¼ cup fresh orange juice, and 2 teaspoons *Chia Gel* (page 157)

DAY 17

Breakfast
(400 calories)

Frittata, Raspberry-Topped Yogurt, and English Muffin (V)
1 serving *California Frittata* (page 160)
1 6-ounce container plain fat-free Smári Icelandic yogurt or Greek yogurt topped with ½ cup fresh or frozen, thawed raspberries and sprinkled with ½ teaspoon chia seeds and, if desired, 1 teaspoon honey or agave nectar
½ whole grain gluten-free or sprouted-grain English muffin, toasted, with 1 teaspoon almond butter

Lunch
(550 calories)

Turkey Wrap and Arugula Salad
1 large whole grain gluten-free wrap or sprouted-grain tortilla stuffed with 2½ ounces smoked turkey breast, ⅛ cup sliced red onion, 1 cup baby arugula, and 1 tablespoon honey mustard
2 cups baby arugula salad with 12 red seedless grapes, 1 ounce crumbled soft goat cheese, 1 tablespoon sliced almonds, 2 teaspoons extra-virgin olive oil, and apple cider vinegar to taste

Dinner
(550 calories)

Curried Turkey Burger, Quinoa, and Red Peppers
1 serving *Indian-Spiced Turkey Burgers with Chia Curry Ketchup* (page 178)
1 cup cooked quinoa, prepared with 2 teaspoons chia seeds; stir in 1 tablespoon chopped fresh cilantro
1 large sliced red pepper (or 1 sliced zucchini) sautéed with 1 teaspoon unrefined virgin coconut oil
10 red seedless grapes

Snacks (200 calories each)

Edamame with Sea Salt (V)
1 cup cooked edamame in pods with sea salt to taste

Chocolate Raisins (V)
¼ cup chocolate-covered raisins

DAY 18

Breakfast (400 calories)

Tart Cherry and Almond-Topped Cereal (V)
1¼ cups whole grain gluten-free cereal flakes with 1 cup fat-free milk with 3 tablespoons dried tart cherries and 1 tablespoon sliced almonds

Lunch (550 calories)

Tuna Salad Platter
1 serving *Mediterranean Tuna Salad* (page 164)
20 small gluten-free whole grain crackers, such as Mary's Gone Crackers
½ cup hummus with 2 medium celery stalks

Dinner (550 calories)

Veggie Stir-Fry with Ginger Rice (V)
1 cup each fresh broccoli florets and sliced cremini or white button mushrooms and 4 ounces extra-firm tofu stir-fried in 2 teaspoons sesame oil and tossed with 1 tablespoon all-natural kung pao or stir-fry sauce
1 cup steamed brown rice or wild rice with 1 teaspoon freshly grated ginger and 1 teaspoon chia seeds

Snacks (200 calories each)

Pear with Cheese (V)
1 pear, cut into wedges, with 1 ounce blue cheese or aged goat cheese

Crackers and Dip (V)
1 serving *Chia Edamame Dip* (page 188) with 13 small whole grain gluten-free crackers, such as Mary's Gone Crackers

DAY 19

Breakfast (400 calories)

Egg Muffin Sandwich (V)
1 egg "fried" in a cooking spray–coated nonstick skillet and served in a toasted whole grain gluten-free or sprouted-grain hamburger bun or English muffin with a 1-ounce slice of part-skim mozzarella cheese, 1 large slice of tomato, and ½ cup fresh baby arugula tossed with ½ teaspoon of lemon juice
¾ cup cubed mango or other fruit

Lunch (550 calories)	**Citrus Rice Salad with Chicken** 1 serving *Orange-Chia Rice Salad with Fresh Mint* (page 169) 4 ounces boneless, skinless pregrilled chicken breast or 1 rotisserie chicken breast with skin, reheated in a microwave if necessary 1 cup 1% low-sodium cottage cheese (or ½ cup part-skim ricotta cheese) with 1 teaspoon each roasted sunflower seeds and honey or agave nectar
Dinner (550 calories)	**Turkey Burger with Broccoli Soup and Baked Potato** 4 ounces lean ground chicken burger or turkey burger and 1 large, thick slice of red onion, grilled or pan cooked, topped with a ¾-ounce slice of Swiss cheese and fresh rosemary to taste; served without a bun 1 serving *Broccoli Velvet Soup* (page 183) 1 small baked potato with 2 teaspoons sour cream and sea salt to taste
Snacks (200 calories each)	**Almonds (V)** 25 raw almonds **Chips and Salsa (V)** 14 blue or yellow corn tortilla chips with a mixture of ¼ cup salsa and 1 tablespoon *Chia Gel* (page 157)

DAY 20

Breakfast (400 calories)	**Granola and Grapefruit (V)** 1 serving *Chia Granola* (page 159) with ½ cup low-fat (1%) milk or plant-based milk ½ large pink grapefruit with 1 teaspoon honey or agave nectar
Lunch (550 calories)	**Baja Bean Salad with Corn Tortilla (V)** 2 cups mixed baby salad greens tossed with ¾ cup pinto or black beans, 1 medium chopped green pepper (or 1 cup sliced white button mushrooms), ⅔ cup frozen, thawed corn, 1 ounce (¼ cup) shredded or cubed Monterey Jack cheese, 3 tablespoons salsa mixed with 1 tablespoon *Chia Gel* (page 157) and 1 teaspoon extra-virgin olive oil, lime juice, and fresh cilantro to taste 2 6-inch soft corn tortillas
Dinner (550 calories)	**Lentils and Kale with Rice (V)** 1 serving *Coriander Lentils and Kale* (page 184) 1 cup steamed brown basmati rice or millet with 3 tablespoons toasted sliced almonds, lemon wedge, and sea salt to taste

Snacks (200 calories each)	**Crackers and Dip (V)** 1 serving *Chia Edamame Dip* (page 188) with 13 small whole grain gluten-free crackers, such as Mary's Gone Crackers **Brie and Grapes (V)** 1 1½-ounce wedge of Brie cheese with 18 red seedless grapes

DAY 21

Breakfast (400 calories)	**Orange Smoothie Breakfast (V)** 1¼ cups low-fat vanilla yogurt blended into a smoothie with ⅔ cup each fresh orange juice and low-fat (1%) milk (or plant-based milk), 2 tablespoons *Chia Gel* (page 157), and about 3 large ice cubes
Lunch (550 calories)	**Double Salad Lunch (V)** 1 serving *Chia Caesar Kale Salad* (page 170) ¾ cup cannellini or other white beans tossed with 1 teaspoon each extra-virgin olive oil and balsamic vinegar (or lemon juice) and fresh herbs to taste 1 1-ounce whole grain gluten-free or sprouted-grain roll 1 cup red or green seedless grapes
Dinner (550 calories)	**Chicken Burger with Broccoli Soup and Baked Potato** 4 ounces lean ground chicken burger or turkey burger and 1 large, thick slice of red onion, grilled or pan cooked, topped with a ¾-ounce slice of Swiss cheese and fresh rosemary to taste; served without a bun 1 serving *Broccoli Velvet Soup* (page 183) 1 small baked potato with 2 teaspoons sour cream and sea salt to taste
Snacks (200 calories each)	**Apple and Pistachios (V)** 1 small apple and 35 roasted or salt-and-pepper pistachios **Deviled Eggs (V)** 1 hard-boiled egg, halved, yolk mixed with 2 teaspoons vegan mayonnaise and a pinch of cayenne pepper 15 baby carrots

DAY 22

Breakfast (400 calories)	**Banana- and Walnut-Topped Cereal (V)** 1¼ cups whole grain gluten-free cereal flakes with 1 cup fat-free milk (or plant-based milk), 1 small sliced banana, 1½ teaspoons chopped walnuts, and 2 teaspoons chia seeds

Lunch (550 calories)	**Veggie Sandwich and White Bean Salad (V)** 2 slices whole grain gluten-free bread stuffed with ½ cup each sliced roasted bell pepper (or sliced grilled zucchini) and thinly sliced cucumber, 2 thin slices red onion, ½ cup fresh baby arugula, 1½ ounces soft goat cheese, and 1 teaspoon each extra-virgin olive oil and balsamic vinegar ¾ cup cannellini or other white beans tossed with 1 teaspoon each extra-virgin olive oil, balsamic vinegar, and chia seeds; add fresh herbs to taste
Dinner (550 calories)	**Egg Tostada Stack with Dinner Sausage** 1 serving *Veggie Tostada Stack with Egg and Avocado* (page 180) 1 (3-ounce) link gluten-free poultry sausage, such as Applegate Organics Chicken & Apple Sausage ½ cup mango cubes or other fruit
Snacks (200 calories each)	**Apple with Almond Butter (V)** 1 small apple cut into wedges with 4 teaspoons almond butter **Cookie Break (V)** 1 cookie *Chia White Chocolate Macadamia Cookies* (page 190)

DAY 23

Breakfast (400 calories)	**Almond Butter and Banana Toastie (V)** 2 slices whole grain gluten-free bread filled with 1½ tablespoons almond butter, ½ teaspoon chia seeds, and ½ sliced small banana; toast in cooking spray–coated skillet or panini press ½ small banana
Lunch (550 calories)	**Basmati Salad with Swiss-Turkey Rolls** 1 serving *Dill Roasted Carrot and Basmati Salad* (page 172) 2 1-ounce slices of deli roasted or smoked turkey, each rolled up with a ¾-ounce slice of Swiss cheese and ½ teaspoon Dijon mustard; secure each with a toothpick 1 small apple
Dinner (550 calories)	**Chicken Pesto Pasta with Peppers** 1½ cups cooked whole grain gluten-free spaghetti tossed with 2 tablespoons each pesto sauce and *Chia Gel* (page 157), 3 ounces shredded rotisserie chicken breast meat, ½ thinly sliced fresh red pepper (or ½ cup gently steamed sliced zucchini), and ½ minced serrano pepper

Snacks (200 calories each)	**Cheesy Corn Tortilla with Guacamole (V)** 1 6-inch soft corn tortilla with 2 tablespoons shredded Monterey Jack cheese, warmed; serve with 1 serving *Chia Guacamole* (page 189) or 3 tablespoons other guacamole on the side **Mango Chia Yogurt (V)** ¾ cup low-fat vanilla yogurt topped with ½ cup cubed mango or banana and ½ teaspoon chia seeds

DAY 24

Breakfast (400 calories)	**Blueberry Pancakes and Yogurt (V)** 1 serving *Blueberry Buckwheat Pancakes* (page 162) 1 6-ounce container plain fat-free Smári Icelandic yogurt or Greek yogurt drizzled with 1½ tablespoons chopped walnuts or pistachios, 1 teaspoon chia seeds, and, if desired, 1 teaspoon honey or agave nectar
Lunch (550 calories)	**Bagel Deli Melt and Cup of Soup** ½ (2-ounce portion) whole grain gluten-free bagel topped with 1 teaspoon Dijon mustard, 2 ounces lean ham or smoked turkey, and a 1-ounce slice of Swiss cheese; heat in the microwave until the cheese melts 1 cup reduced-sodium split pea soup (about 180 calories) 15 baby carrots
Dinner (550 calories)	**Fish Tacos and Guacamole** 1 serving *Soft Fish Tacos with Chia Pico de Gallo* (page 175) 1 serving *Chia Guacamole* (page 189) or 3 tablespoons other guacamole ½ cup organic vegetarian refried beans 1 cup mango cubes or other fruit
Snacks (200 calories each)	**Chocolate Pudding (V)** 1 serving *Chia Chocolate Pudding* (page 193), served with 3 large fresh strawberries if desired **Pineapple and Smoked Turkey Skewers** 1½ ounces cubed smoked turkey on skewers with 1½ cups pineapple cubes

DAY 25

Breakfast (400 calories)	**Breakfast Crostini (V)** 1 whole grain gluten-free or sprouted-grain English muffin, split and toasted, each muffin half topped with ⅓ cup part-skim ricotta cheese, ½ peeled and diced kiwi fruit, ½ teaspoon honey or agave nectar, ¼ teaspoon chia seeds, and sea salt to taste

Lunch (550 calories)	**Thai Peanut Noodles and Orange (V)** 1 serving *Thai Tofu Peanut Chia Noodles* (page 165) 1 large orange 10 raw almonds
Dinner (550 calories)	**Roasted Turkey with Beet and Goat Cheese Salad** 1 serving *Beet and Goat Cheese Salad* (page 185) 5 ounces turkey tenderloin brushed with 1 tablespoon horseradish or Dijon mustard and roasted at 400°F until well done, about 25 minutes; season with sea salt to taste 1 large baked sweet potato, sprinkled with 1 ounce crumbled soft goat cheese, 1 teaspoon chia seeds, and fresh basil to taste
Snacks (200 calories each)	**Snack Mix (V)** ⅓ cup snack mix (dried fruit, nuts, and seeds) OR 1 (3.5-ounce) Mamma Chia Chia Squeeze Vitality Snack + 3 tablespoons snack mix **Frozen Yogurt Sundae (V)** ¾ cups fat-free mint or vanilla frozen yogurt or plant-based frozen dessert drizzled with mixture of 2 teaspoons each *Chia Gel* (page 157) and organic chocolate syrup

DAY 26

Breakfast (400 calories)	**Oatmeal and Turkey Bacon** 1 serving *Steel-Cut "Superfood" Oatmeal* (page 158) 1 ounce nitrite-free turkey bacon, such as Applegate Organics Uncured Turkey Bacon ½ large pink grapefruit with 1 teaspoon honey or agave nectar or 2 kiwi fruits
Lunch (550 calories)	**Sushi and Fruit** 12-piece brown rice California sushi (from market or restaurant) with tamari soy sauce, pickled ginger, and wasabi paste to taste ½ large pink grapefruit with 1 teaspoon honey or agave nectar or 2 kiwi fruits
Dinner (550 calories)	**Caprese Spaghetti with Leafy Grape Salad (V)** 1 cup cooked whole grain gluten-free spaghetti tossed with 2 ounces cubed part-skim mozzarella cheese, 1 diced medium tomato, 2 tablespoons chopped fresh basil, 1 minced garlic clove, 1½ teaspoons extra-virgin olive oil, and sea salt to taste 2 cups mixed baby salad greens with 8 red seedless grapes and 1½ teaspoons each extra-virgin olive oil, balsamic vinegar, and chia seeds

<table>
<tr>
<td rowspan="2">Snacks
(200 calories each)</td>
<td>

Chips and Salsa (V)

14 blue or yellow corn tortilla chips with mixture of ¼ cup salsa and 1 tablespoon *Chia Gel* (page 157)

</td>
</tr>
<tr>
<td>

Dark Chocolate (V)

1¼-ounce portion dark chocolate bar (at least 60% cacao) or 4 Dagoba Organic New Moon Bittersweet Dark Chocolate squares

</td>
</tr>
</table>

DAY 27

<table>
<tr>
<td>Breakfast
(400 calories)</td>
<td>

Mexican Breakfast Scramble (V)

Scramble 1 egg, 2 tablespoons *Chia Gel* (page 157), and 12 grape tomatoes in a cooking spray–coated nonstick skillet and stir in 6 blue or yellow corn tortilla chips and 1 ounce (¼ cup) shredded Monterey Jack cheese; serve with 2 tablespoons salsa and 1 serving *Chia Guacamole* (page 189) or 3 tablespoons other guacamole on the side

</td>
</tr>
<tr>
<td>Lunch
(550 calories)</td>
<td>

Chicken Salad with Grapes

1 serving *Green Tea Chicken and Grape Salad* (page 168)
20 small gluten-free crackers, such as Mary's Gone Crackers
1 cup red or green seedless grapes

</td>
</tr>
<tr>
<td>Dinner
(550 calories)</td>
<td>

Lentils and Kale with Rice (V)

1 serving *Coriander Lentils and Kale* (page 184)
1 cup steamed brown basmati rice or millet with 3 tablespoons toasted sliced almonds, lemon wedge, and salt to taste

</td>
</tr>
<tr>
<td rowspan="2">Snacks
(200 calories each)</td>
<td>

Chia Cherry Vanilla Smoothie (V)

1 serving *Chia Cherry Vanilla Smoothie* (page 191)

</td>
</tr>
<tr>
<td>

Shrimp Cocktail and Mamma Chia

10 large cooked chilled shrimp with 1½ tablespoons cocktail sauce; serve with 1 (10-ounce) bottle Mamma Chia Vitality Beverage or 1 (5-ounce) glass wine

</td>
</tr>
</table>

DAY 28

<table>
<tr>
<td>Breakfast
(400 calories)</td>
<td>

Bagel with Scallion Cream Cheese (V)

1 4-ounce toasted whole grain gluten-free or sprouted-grain bagel with 2 tablespoons Neufchâtel (light cream cheese) sprinkled with 1 minced scallion

</td>
</tr>
</table>

Lunch (550 calories)	**Pear and Goat Cheese Salad with Chicken** 1 serving *Mesclun Salad with Pear, Walnuts, and Goat Cheese* (page 173) 2 pregrilled boneless, skinless chicken thighs, warm or chilled (about 4 ounces each)
Dinner (550 calories)	**Egg Tostada Stack with Dinner Sausage** 1 serving *Veggie Tostada Stack with Egg and Avocado* (page 180) 1 3-ounce link gluten-free poultry sausage, such as Applegate Organics Chicken & Apple Sausage ½ cup mango cubes or other fruit
Snacks (200 calories each)	**Pineapple and Smoked Turkey Skewers** 1½ ounces cubed smoked turkey on skewers with 1½ cups pineapple cubes **Pear with Cheese (V)** 1 pear, cut into wedges, with 1 ounce blue cheese or aged goat cheese

DAY 29

Breakfast (400 calories)	**Yogurt with Strawberry Jam and Almonds (V)** 1 cup plain fat-free Smári Icelandic yogurt or Greek yogurt topped with 1 serving *Fresh Strawberry–Chia Seed Jam* (page 161) 20 raw almonds 1 small banana
Lunch (550 calories)	**Turkey and Avocado Sandwich with Carrots and Hummus** 1 whole grain gluten-free or sprouted-grain hamburger bun stuffed with ½ sliced Hass avocado, 3 ounces smoked turkey breast, 1 large slice red onion, ½ cup baby arugula, and 2 teaspoons Dijon mustard 10 baby carrots with ¼ cup hummus or 1% low-sodium cottage cheese
Dinner (550 calories)	**Salmon with Veggie Fried Rice** 5 ounces pan-grilled wild salmon or other fish, spritzed with olive oil cooking spray and sprinkled with sea salt and freshly ground black pepper to taste 1 serving *Thai Basil Veggie Fried Rice* (page 186)
Snacks (200 calories each)	**Apple and Pistachios (V)** 1 small apple and 35 roasted or salt-and-pepper pistachios **Frozen Yogurt Sundae (V)** ¾ cups fat-free mint or vanilla frozen yogurt or plant-based frozen dessert drizzled with a mixture of 2 teaspoons each *Chia Gel* (page 157) and organic chocolate syrup

DAY 30

Breakfast (400 calories)	**Cinnamon Toast, Grapefruit, and Vanilla Milk (V)** 1 slice whole grain gluten-free or sprouted-grain toast spread with 1 teaspoon butter or vegan butter and sprinkled with ½ teaspoon honey or agave nectar and a pinch of cinnamon ½ large pink grapefruit with 1 teaspoon honey or agave nectar 1 cup almond or other plant-based vanilla milk 15 raw almonds
Lunch (550 calories)	**Tropical Quinoa and Kale with Soup (V)** 1 serving *Tropical Quinoa and Kale* (page 66) 1½ cups low-sodium black bean or other soup (about 200 calories) 20 grape tomatoes, halved and tossed with 1 teaspoon extra-virgin olive oil and sea salt to taste
Dinner (550 calories)	**Sausage and "Fries"** 1 3-ounce link gluten-free poultry sausage, such as Applegate Organics Chicken & Apple Sausage, served on whole grain gluten-free or sprouted-grain frankfurter bun with 2 teaspoons each ketchup, Dijon mustard, and minced red onion 1 serving *Chia–Sweet Potato "Fries"* (page 179) 1 cup steamed baby spinach or zucchini, lemon wedge, and sea salt to taste 1 cup almond or other plant-based vanilla milk
Snacks (200 calories each)	**Chocolate Pudding (V)** 1 serving *Chia Chocolate Pudding* (page 193), served with 3 large fresh strawberries if desired **Mango Chia Yogurt (V)** ¾ cup low-fat vanilla yogurt topped with ½ cup cubed mango or banana and ½ teaspoon chia seeds

SEEDS OF WISDOM

Food should be fun.

—THOMAS KELLER, *chef and author*

5

·······

MOVING INTO VITALITY

N ot long ago I was at my local gym, and as I was working out I observed a group of women exercising together. The one who really caught my eye was clearly the oldest of the bunch, but only her beautiful silver hair gave her away. She was doing crunches and lunges like nobody's business—really kind of running circles around the other gals. Her body was lean and her muscles enviably well defined. She had a joyful bounce in her step and an enchanting smile on her face. She radiated vitality. *Wow,* I thought, *what's* her *secret?*

I later learned that that delightful dynamo in the gym was eighty-three and also practices yoga and does ballroom dancing. She loves to paint, sells her hand-painted greeting cards, and has a diverse community circle. So, along with physical activity, she leads a rich, full life; she probably has good genes as well. But I still can't help but think that her exercise habits play a big role in how energetic she is. There's no denying that people who move their bodies on a regular basis have the inside edge when it comes to strength and vitality—and not only in attaining strength and vitality, but in sustaining it. My mother-in-law, who is also eighty-three, is a real live wire, and I can't help but think that part of it is owing to the fact that she's still out there playing tennis three times a week.

I don't have to tell you how many more years you'll live if you habitually work out, or fill you in on how much lower your risk of about a hundred and one diseases will be if you just take a brisk walk every morning. You already know that exercise is good for you. What sometimes gets lost in the message, though, is just how vibrant and energetic you can feel when you're regularly moving your body— not only physically, but emotionally, mentally, and even spiritually. It's another spoke in the wheel of attaining vitality. There's a bit of a paradox, there, I know: you need to already *have* energy to get out there and exercise to create more energy. But the tipping point is very low. You really don't need to expend much effort to start feeling the rewards. And you've got chia to help you get over the hump!

Some of you, I suspect, got over that hump a long time ago and are already passionate about exercise. Given that chia helps power some of the best runners on the planet, many exercise enthusiasts are already fans of the seeds; maybe you're one of them and just picked up this book to see how to work more of that perfect workout fuel into your life. Or maybe you're one of the 40 percent of people who are sitting out physical activity entirely because you don't have the time to make it a priority in your life. Or maybe you're a serial exerciser—someone who avidly adopts a workout routine, lets it fall by the wayside, then does the same thing all over again—repeatedly. Whatever your scenario, I think it's useful to step back and ask, *Hey, what am I doing (or not doing) and why? Can I improve the way I think about and experience exercise?* No matter what your base level is, I believe you can.

The one thing I don't like about fitness imperatives is the guilt factor. All the public messages designed to get people moving are important and necessary, but they can create inner turmoil that's often self-defeating. If you're not doing anything at all, you feel guilty. If you're not doing enough, you feel guilty. If you've lapsed, you feel guilty. Even triathletes, who are surely doing more than their share of exercise, torment themselves if they miss a workout. I, for one, am against exercise-induced guilt! Being able to move your body is a gift, and when you're in the groove, moving should feel absolutely wonderful. But it's my observation that we put too much pressure on ourselves—pressure to engage in a certain kind of exercise, pressure to work out a particular amount of time, pressure to work out at a specific intensity, or pressure to use exercise exclusively as a way of losing weight. All this makes exercise become just another thing that we're not doing "right," a stressor rather than the joyful, life-affirming undertaking it can be. Maybe that's why so many people run away from the chance to improve their health and vitality.

On these next few pages, I'll explore a few different ways of thinking about exercise with the goal of helping you find physical activity that not only helps you be healthy, lean, and strong but engages your mind and soul, too. And for those of you who've already found your perfect routine? I think there's value in evaluating your approach to working out and asking whether you're getting all the vitality-boosting benefits from exercise that you can.

My go-to workout is yoga, and in the appendix to this book, I'll introduce you to the *Chia Vitality* yoga practice. I consider yoga a spiritual practice—how nice that it also helps you whip your body into shape! Yoga, you might say, brings your whole being into harmony. The beauty of yoga, too, is that it can be what you want it to be. It's malleable, so no matter what your body is telling you, there's a yoga practice to match. By including a routine here (and one that you can refine to satisfy your own body's cravings), I want to give you a low-pressure practice that's like having a health safety net—always there for you wherever you go, whenever you need it.

HOW EXERCISE ENHANCES VITALITY

It's a mood lifter. The power of physical activity to trigger chemicals associated with state of mind, pleasure, and pain reduction has put exercise on the list of remedies for depression. Study after study has found that not only does exercise relieve symptoms of depression, it also helps prevent them from reoccurring.

It sharpens thinking. A session on the elliptical isn't going to turn you into Albert Einstein, but it can help you stay on the ball and fight off the effects of aging. For years now, researchers at the University of Illinois at Urbana-Champaign have been studying what happens to the brains of older people when they participate in a regular walking program. And in each of the many studies, researchers found improvement. Take the 2010 one where they looked at the brains of people ages fifty-nine to eighty with high-resolution brain imaging after a year of walking. The result? The exercisers had increased brain connectivity and improved scores on cognitive tests. There's proof, too, that you can benefit even if you're not at the age when brain function begins to be a worry. Reviewing studies on exercise and cognition in young adults, New Zealand researchers concluded that regular workouts improve executive functioning—the ability to organize, strategize, pay attention, and remember details.

It boosts creativity. I know this to be true just through my own experience, and maybe you do, too: some of the best ideas come to me while I'm walking or engaged in some other kind of heart-pumping activity. This hypothesis has also been put to the test by researchers who had exercisers engage in either a gentle form of aerobic dance or a faster and more energetic series of aerobic exercises, then measured their creative thinking. Both groups had higher measures of creativity than a similar group who watched a video instead of working out.

LISTENING TO YOUR BODY

If you exercise regularly now or have tried to do so in the past, what drives your choices? Is it something outside yourself, or is it what feels right for your body? I ask because I believe it's all too easy to get caught up in thinking that you have to conform to certain exercise parameters. When many people think about exercise, they imagine that it only counts if they take a giant leap onto the workout-of-the-moment bandwagon even if every cell in their body is disagreeing. Everybody you know swears by spin class? You're on that bike panting and trying to ignore the fact that your back is killing you, you can't see because there's so much sweat in your eyes, and you feel like a mess for the rest of the day. Everybody's into CrossFit, the superintense strength and conditioning program springing up all over the country? You endure it, despite finding that it never makes you feel good, even when it's over. Zumba, you hear, is so much fun? You tag along with your friends each week even though it makes you feel like a clod because you are naturally rhythmically challenged.

Listen, I know there's always some level of discomfort with exercise. The only way that the body gets stronger is by facing a challenge, then building itself up to be better at that particular type of movement the next time. And, of course, you can't just do it once and get the benefits; you've got to keep at it. But that's exactly why it's so important to pay attention to what your body is telling you. If you choose a workout because you think you should do it even while your body is saying, *No I shouldn't!*, you're eventually going to give it up and, more than likely, end up doing nothing at all.

Listening to your body also means heeding its rhythms and cycles. This is something that avid exercisers might especially want to consider, since it's easy to get into a workout routine that doesn't let up—even when it should. When your body is up for the challenge of a long run, a monster hike, or an hour of hilly cycling, go for it! But also respect that there will be other times when your body is asking for a restorative form of movement like some yoga, simple stretching, or a slow stroll around the block. Just on practical terms, this is one way to avoid injury. Bodies need downtime! For those of you who find yourself in a stop-and-start relationship with exercise, clueing in on what your body needs at different times can also help you stay committed to physical activity. You'll love movement so much more if you heed your body's needs.

As someone who spent years on a roller-coaster ride of health difficulties, I put a lot of faith in listening to what the body has to say. When I was in remission from my autoimmune struggles, vigorous exercise felt wonderful. I got all the benefits: improved mood; greater strength, flexibility, and balance; better posture; more stamina; and a good night's sleep (one of exercise's great but unsung gifts). But I also know that if I had guilted myself into vigorous exercise during those times when my body was fragile, it could have compromised my health even more *and* colored my attitude toward working out—instead of associating it with making me feel good, I would have associated it with making me feel bad. So I took the literal path of least resistance: I heeded what my body was telling me and found ways to move in fairly undemanding ways—*but I did move*. And it was a revelation! I got nearly as many benefits as I did with the vigorous exercise. I felt better, and I never dreaded or outright hated physical activity.

Listening to your body takes some practice. Sometimes fatigue and lethargy (especially when you haven't been moving much at all) indicate that your body needs to work up a sweat, not take a break. There can be some value in overriding your body a bit, if you're doing it within reason. Distracting yourself from mild discomfort with some music that rocks your world or reruns on a TV set up in front of a treadmill can be enough to help you stick with exercise without compromising your body's needs. Exercise increases blood flow, which means your cells get more of the nutrients and oxygen they need to produce more energy. Talk about a wake-up call! Give yourself a test: take a walk around the block and see if you don't feel better immediately. If you do, that can be a sign that you need to walk or exercise otherwise more.

If, however, you're the type who sticks to a somewhat punishing exercise schedule no matter what, your challenge may be to put the fears and guilt you feel on mute while you check in with yourself. Typical signs of overdoing it are sore muscles for more than two days, getting sick more often, an elevated heart rate, fatigue, insomnia, and depression. Whether your might be over- or underdoing it, ask yourself, *What do I need in this moment?* That's the operative question for everyone.

SEEDS OF WISDOM

· ·

All truly great thoughts are conceived while walking.

—FRIEDRICH NIETZSCHE, *German philosopher*

And it's a question the chia-based diet in this book can help you answer. When you're eating foods that nourish and energize you, it's easier to be attuned to your body. Part of this, I believe, is just psychological. Eating well gives you a sense of what it's like to feel well, and that can make you want to improve other aspects of your lifestyle. Plus when you're going to the trouble of eating consciously, you don't want your exercise habits (or lack thereof) to cancel out the benefits of your healthy eating habits. Let chia lead you down the path of paying closer attention to your body's needs.

THE SEED FOR SPEED

In his charming self-deprecating way, Jeff Ford will be the first to tell you that he's not a fast runner. His lack of speed, in fact, was a favorite topic of a running partner, who liked to tease him about his lackluster pace while the two of them were training for a half marathon. When the day finally came, though, the situation switched. "It was *me* pushing her to go faster, not the other way around," remembers Jeff, forty-one, who lives in Long Beach, California. His speed also increased each mile—"which was not indicative of my usual pace," he says. Finally, by mile 8, his training partner told him to go ahead, and he did, finishing the race twenty-five minutes ahead of her. "What the hell got into you this morning?" she asked.

Chia seeds, of course.

Like a lot of runners, Jeff had heard all about how the Tarahumara Indians used chia to power them through their long runs. A close friend—"the source of all things alternative in my life," he says—had clued him in several years before chia appeared on the greater population's radar, and he began mixing it with water (3 parts water to 1 part chia) and a little agave for a morning boost. But he had never experimented with the seeds on a race day until that fateful half marathon. "I had a big bowl of chia mixed with water and fruit that morning," says Jeff, an adjunct professor of economics at the University of San Francisco School of Management and director of sales operations for truecar.com. "It gave me amazing sustained energy. When my training partner asked what got into me, I said, 'I don't know, but I feel like a machine!'" Last year, chia sustained him through the seventy-mile Ironman triathlon in Hawaii, too.

The seeds are still a daily addition to Jeff's diet. "I have a sensitive stomach and some gluten sensitivity, so I'm really cautious about what I eat, but chia never bothers me, and I feel good about eating something with so many antioxidants and other nutrients," he says. He's converted his fiancée into a chia believer, too. They now both start the day with what they call "crazy toast": gluten-free rice bread for him, regular whole-grain for her, each topped with peanut butter, fruit—and chia seeds.

THE PLEASURE PRINCIPLE

One thing that the body needs for sure is pleasure. If you're lucky enough to get into the flow while exercising—a term coined by psychologist Mihály Csikszentmihályi to describe the state of heightened awareness of the body and full immersion in the present moment—your workout will feel good. You may even feel "high." If you've never felt the connection between moving and bliss and instead always emerge from the gym feeling overtaxed and like a huffing, puffing mess, it may be because you're working out according to a set of prescribed rules that simply don't jibe with your DNA.

That, at least, is what some exercise experts are beginning to think accounts for the differences between people who get giddy at the idea of working up a sweat and those who'd rather drink castor oil than go for a two-mile run. A series of studies led by Panteleimon Ekkekakis, PhD, a professor of kinesiology at Iowa State University, has shown that the point where exercise begins to feel bad varies widely. Some people find that pushing to what's called their ventilatory threshold— the intensity at which you're working so hard it becomes difficult to talk—is pleasurable, while others find it decidedly unpleasant. The trouble is, the lower threshold group often push beyond their limits, perhaps adhering to recommendations that set the bar higher than suits their bodies' natural abilities. Those difficult and perhaps even painful sessions breed contempt for exercise, and ultimately the routine gets tossed out the window.

This research shows that exercise is very forgiving if you are able to do it in a way that suits your body. So what if you're not going to cycle a century (a hundred-mile bike ride) like your next-door neighbor? Perhaps you weren't born that way! Swimming for forty-five minutes may be more your speed, and the benefits will be appreciable. This isn't to say that you shouldn't set fitness goals that seem above your capabilities now. The improvement of your lung capacity, the increased ability of your heart to pump more oxygen to your working muscles, and the bump up in strength that comes from repeatedly challenging your body can all help make what you find so difficult today much easier down the road. You've seen those seventy-five-year-olds competing in marathons for the first time. People can take up physical challenges and surprise everybody, including themselves. This is where vitality can lead you.

Some research also suggests that all's well that ends well. Dr. Ekkekakis's lab did a study with thirty-one men and women who were far from exercise enthusiasts, which is to say they had very low levels of activity. The group was asked to get on treadmills and walk at an intensity that was 10 percent above the level where they felt comfortable. In one session, they simply stopped at the end of twenty minutes;

in a second session, they cooled down for 5 minutes. When later asked which exercise session they'd repeat, a majority went for the session that ended with an easy cooldown.

The impetus for this study sprang from research showing that if an event ends well, it will be remembered well—despite what happened in most of its duration. And this theory worked for many of the exercise study participants: because the cooldown made them feel good, they viewed that session as one they'd try again. This idea is a good one, although it is by no means new. Yogis have been ending yoga sessions with *savasana*—the act of lying in repose for five minutes or more—for ages, and it works to cement fond feelings for yoga nearly every time.

FALL IN LOVE WITH EXERCISE

There are all kinds of tricks you can employ to help you stay motivated to exercise. But rather than teach you how to fool yourself into sticking with an exercise routine, I want to talk about what I believe is the best way to stay inspired: Fall in love with moving your body. Even though exercise has inherent vitality-enhancing qualities, if you hate every weight you lift, every downward dog you angle your body into, or every jog around the block you take, you're not going to stick with it, no matter how many tricks you employ. If it's fun and feels good, you're going to keep doing it. Simple as that.

Both the bane and the beauty of physical activity is that it's highly individual: the bane, because wouldn't it be easy if there were just one thing everyone could do for health; the beauty, because there's choice! And variety! There are so many ways to move your body that I'm confident you're going to find the one that suits you. You may even discover that, with the right activity, exercise becomes a very deep, soulful experience. My own experience has been that movement allows the mind to enter a very contemplative and serene state, allowing for a sense of peace and union. Unity and creativity happen side by side. Plus, when you keep an open mind and become better attuned to activities that nurture you physically, emotionally, mentally, and spiritually, you create a practice that brings you closer to true vitality.

Finding your dream workout is going to take some trial and error and perhaps a little adventurousness on your part, but you will succeed. Here are five ways to fall in love.

1. Ask a friend for an introduction.

Sometimes a particular type of exercise *sounds* interesting, but giving it a try on your own can be a little daunting. The next time a friend regales you with tales about outrigger canoeing or single-scull rowing, ballroom dance classes or cardio barre workouts, stand-up paddleboarding, stadium stair climbing, Pilates mat sessions, or yoga set to music—anything that captures your imagination—ask him or her to take you along or help introduce you to the beginner's version. Most aficionados love to recruit others, and it's good to have a buddy you can talk to about the finer points of your (hopefully!) newfound passion. If you don't know anybody who already practices your dream activity on a regular basis, invite somebody to try something new with you! You won't be the only beginner, and even if you don't like the activity, it will be a good bonding experience.

2. Go on your own fact-finding mission.

I tried it; I didn't like it. Fair enough. If you try an exercise class or a particular activity and it just doesn't speak to you, there is no reason you should continue. But before you write it off, I would ask you, just how deeply did you dive into it? Say you decide to try spinning, so you go to a spinning class at a local studio. Turns out, the music's annoying, the instructor even more so, and the intensity of the class over the top. But that's *one* class; others may be entirely different. This is especially true for any class-based exercise you could try, but really any type of exercise will vary depending on the conditions—and your mood. Do yourself the favor of really shopping around before you decide a workout isn't for you. There are so many variables that make a workout either pleasurable or unpleasant that it really pays to check something out from several angles.

3. Join a workout group.

Along the same lines as #1, exercising with like-minded people can turn workouts into an entirely different experience from going it alone. When people walk, swim, cycle, run, paddle, kick a soccer ball—the list goes on—as a group, the camaraderie they develop is truly unique. And when you join a workout group, it's another way of expanding your world, as I talk about in chapter 7. (Talk about killing two birds with one stone!) There are some well-established groups for adult exercisers (you don't necessarily have to be really good at the sport); for example, if you like being in the water, you could check out a group like U.S. Masters Swimming, which provides coached workouts in the pool. Whatever your workout of choice, you can find less formal, locally grown groups of people who just get together at a specific time. Check bulletin boards in local sports stores and meetup.com, which helps you find (or start) a workout group in your area.

4. Train for something.

As with just about anything, having a goal in sight can steady your interest and, when the job is done, make you feel pretty darn awesome! Don't let the notion that you've never competed or engaged in organized sports stop you. You can train for something as simple as a five-kilometer (about three miles) walk. It can be particularly inspiring to train for an event that raises money for a fund you believe in—a swim to help inner-city kids get into the pool, for instance, or an indoor cycling ride to raise money for breast cancer. There are literally hundreds of options.

5. Put on your walking shoes.

This is the back-to-basics workout: our bodies were made for walking. I ask you, what could be simpler? If nothing else sticks, walking is a great way to boost your fitness quotient. It's incredibly effective, healthwise, with a low rate of injury, and can't be beat for convenience. If it's boring to you, grab a friend or family member, make a phone call, listen to a mystery novel on your iPod as you move (you'll want to walk just to find out what happens next), window-shop, or find a spot with lots of greenery and trees—that's my personal favorite. Just do whatever it takes to make it work for you, and don't be surprised if you get hooked within a few days!

SEEDS OF KNOWLEDGE

GREEN YOUR EXERCISE ROUTINE

Even if you don't consider yourself a nature lover, there's evidence that greenery can boost your mood and energy, lower stress, and help safeguard your health. Just looking out a window at a natural landscape has been shown to lower blood pressure and heart rate. Pictures of nature help people recover more quickly from surgery. You can probably see where I'm going with this: taking your workout outdoors may take its benefits to a new level.

I'm all for exercising when and where you can, so if walking on a treadmill instead of in a park is all you can manage, I applaud you for any effort you make. Personally, I find being outside, especially moving among the trees, up a hillside or mountain, or near a lake or ocean, spiritually uplifting. It reminds you that you're connected to the world; you are part of the ecosystem—part of the One Life. And research shows there are real differences when you put nature in your line of sight as you exercise.

In one 2012 study, conducted in England, exercisers cycled while watching a video that simulated riding through a very lush environment. At various times, the video was tinted green, red, or gray. After cycling, the study participants were asked to answer questions about their state of mind. Not only did the greenery put them in a better mood than the other tints, it made them feel as though they weren't working so hard. In Scotland, researchers put portable devices on volunteers to measure their brain waves, then had them walk through three different settings: a historic urban but lightly trafficked shopping district; a green space with trees and playing fields; and a busy commercial district with heavy traffic. Not surprisingly, the walkers' levels of arousal and frustration dropped as soon as they hit the green zone, and they entered a more reflective, meditative state.

These, I believe, are things we know intuitively. Think of exercising outdoors, where your gaze can fall on the natural beauty (even if it's just in an urban park or waterfront—or a window looking out!), as a gift you can give yourself.

ACKNOWLEDGING THE EBBS AND FLOWS

Exercise is one of those areas where you have to have compassion for yourself. As with just about anything, there may be times when life requires that you let exercise slide. But if you've taken the time to find one (or more) activities that you love and have established a routine for multiple days of the week, you'll be able to pick it up again when things settle down.

Those early days of Mamma Chia found me putting in days that left little room for getting on a yoga mat or taking a walk in the hills. I tried not to beat myself up about it by keeping things in perspective: this, too, I told myself, shall pass! And it did. I got back to yoga and to walking. I got back to strength training, which I feel is so important now that I'm in my forties, the age when you begin to lose muscle in earnest if you don't do something to keep it intact. One thing that helped me restart was sessions with a personal trainer. At first I never told anyone I was seeing a trainer (except my husband, of course!); rightly or wrongly, I had a sense that it was the privileged person's easy way out. But having the help of a trainer was an excellent way for me to reassess where I was so that I didn't just launch back into the same routine I had before my break. The trainer was able to evaluate what I needed at the time and help me ease back into regular workouts.

Training can be affordable if you explore the options. For instance, it doesn't have to be an ongoing relationship; in some cases, you can pay a trainer for a few sessions to help you develop a routine, then continue on your own. It's also possible to buddy up with friends for semi-private sessions, which lowers the cost considerably, and some gyms offer discounted personal training rates if you go at nonpeak hours. There are even online "virtual" trainers.

This is just one option. What's most important is to have confidence that you'll do what's right for your body, and to realize that an "ebb" doesn't mean that you will never "flow" again. Accept the downs, but avoid disparaging yourself for not being as fit as you think you should be (one sure way to get mired in a self-defeating cycle). Just keep treating your body with respect, and know you'll be back on track soon.

THE *CHIA VITALITY* YOGA PRACTICE

I was originally introduced to yoga when I was in my early twenties and in the throes of my autoimmune disorders. I was in a bad state; my body was covered with a rash, and there were many days when dressing myself was so challenging that it was an extreme sport in itself. I simply was not putting much stock in my physical body at the time. I had come seeking instruction on how to flex my spiritual muscles through meditation. My teacher, a lovely Buddhist woman in her fifties, helped me get there through yoga, which was perfect

SEEDS OF WISDOM

Yoga teaches us to cure what need not be endured and endure what cannot be cured.

—B. K. S. IYENGAR, *yoga teacher and founder of Iyengar Yoga*

because it allowed me to move my fragile body in a careful, mindful way while also letting me explore aspects of my spiritual self. (Not a Buddhist myself, I like to say I stand at the heart of all world religions.) This particular initiation into yoga is why I consider it a very spiritual practice, although I know that many people come to it solely for the strength- and flexibility-building benefit it offers. Because the practice of yoga gives you space for contemplation and tools for concentrating the mind and because it promotes nonjudgmental awareness, to me, it offers the best of all worlds. When you do yoga, you are at once developing a fitter body and fostering the alignment to your soul's purpose at the same time.

Another way to look at it is to consider that the poses in yoga are called asanas, which in Sanskrit means "seat." A steady practice of asanas not only enables you to develop balance, flexibility, and strength, it ultimately offers a good "seat" for your soul within your body.

The versatility of yoga is not to be understated. Some people like a very rigorous, intense practice; my body asks for poses that are more soothing, balancing, and restorative. My goal when devising the *Chia Vitality* yoga practice—you'll find the exercises beginning on page 198—was to provide an approximately twenty-five-minute workout that flows gently from one pose to another. It's a confluence of different yoga styles and will definitely get your body heated up, strengthen your muscles, and limber up your joints. You can make it as vigorous or as moderate as you like and shorten or lengthen the practice however you see fit. Some days you may only feel up to doing (or have time for) sun salutations; other days you may want to add more repetitions

LEGS UP THE WALL

I travel a lot, and one of the first things I often do when I get to my hotel room is to lie on the floor and swing my legs up the wall. It's my default position. I can't tell you how many conference calls I've been on where I am angled into an L with my legs upside down (and with no one the wiser on the other end). As yoga poses go, this is a panacea: it's great for calming down and soothing your lower back and tired feet and legs. Trust me, you're going to love it.

LEGS-UP-THE-WALL POSE
Viparita Karani

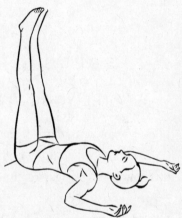

You may want to use one or two (whichever you find most comfort-able) folded blankets, towels, or a bolster for this pose. You can even do it with nothing between you and the floor. I much prefer not to use any props, although I do lay a towel down on the floor if I am in a hotel room.

1. Sit on the floor with one hip against the wall (you'll be turned to the side). Roll onto your back, swivel so that your body is per-pendicular to the wall and, and take your legs up the wall (you'll form an "L"). Press your seat as close to the wall as possible. You may need to wiggle around a bit to get comfortable.
2. Place your arms overhead flat on the floor, bend your elbows to 90 degrees, and breathe.
3. Keep your legs firm without straining. Let your eyes soften or close. Stay in the pose for 5 to 15 minutes.
4. To come out of the pose, bend your knees, push your feet against the wall, and slide off the support. Turn to the side and breathe. Push up with your arms to come to sitting.

to all of the poses. You don't need anything to do the practice other than a few feet of open space. A yoga mat would be nice, too.

If you've never done yoga before, I suggest taking one or more beginner's classes so you can get hands-on help from a teacher. Alternatively, watch instructional videos online so you can really see the poses in action; you can even take classes online through yogaglo.com, which has more than a thousand different classes of all styles and lengths, or view podcasts on the ever-reliable *Yoga Journal* website. You can also just learn by doing. I've provided very detailed instructions including how to sync your breathing with your movements. Give it a try!

SEEDS OF KNOWLEDGE

THE YOGA-VITALITY CONNECTION

You might remember from the initial definition in this book (on page xi) that *vitality* is not one thing, but rather the integration of many—as is yoga. Yoga originated in India about five thousand years ago and comes from a Sanskrit word meaning "to unite." It refers to the union of body, mind, and spirit and the connection between individual consciousness and universal consciousness. Although we've come to know it mostly as a form of exercise, yoga also includes meditation and an overall philosophical outlook that emphasizes love, compassion, and oneness with the world. The ultimate purpose of yoga (in all its forms) is to expand your consciousness and gain a deeper awareness and understanding of your true nature—your soul, that is, and its purpose. For all these reasons, yoga seems particularly compatible with the pursuit of greater vitality. I think you'll find that yoga can improve every aspect of your life, not to mention strengthen your alignment with your own beautiful soul!

6

......

MINDFUL MEDITATION:
A MEANINGFUL "TIME-IN"

f you're like many people I've met along the way, you may have two conflicting reactions to the idea of meditation. On the one hand, you're intrigued. You've heard meditation can make you more relaxed. Who doesn't want relaxation? On the other hand, you've heard that meditation involves trying to sit quietly in an uncomfortable position, watching your belly fill with air, making your mind a complete blank . . . and a lot of other tedious stuff. Have I got it right? If your assumptions are what I just described, I have so much to tell you! Meditation, at least mindful meditation, isn't much like that at all. Most importantly, the benefits you get go way beyond relaxation and stress reduction—that's why instead of calling mindfulness a meaningful "time-out," I like to call it a meaningful "time-in." Mindfulness helps you go deep within yourself and come out more contented, more connected, more grateful, and more compassionate.

I began studying meditation over twenty years ago, originally with a Buddhist teacher, the same one who, you might remember from the previous chapter, introduced me to yoga. The state of my external self, so ravaged from the rashes and hair loss and fatigue, led me to want to cultivate my inner self. I wasn't giving up on my physical body, but I was heeding its clear message: You are more than your physical self. Meditation seemed the right tool at the right time.

It proved to be even more than that. Meditation has had, without a doubt, a great impact on my life. It got me through those rough times when my body would not do what I wanted it to and helped me weather with more grace times when family dynamics were less than delightful. Like chia, meditation is not the single cure for what ails you; but boy can it deliver a feeling of wholeness and vitality! I know of no better way to help you rediscover and connect with your authentic nature and your soul's purpose. So while it's true that meditation can help you achieve a sense of relaxation, it can also fire you up. Just as chia gives you physical energy, meditation also gives you the spiritual, mental, and emotional energy you need to feel dynamic and alive. After studying meditation for many years, I went on to teach it for ten more, instructing groups ranging from 12 to 250 people in private classes, workshops, and corporate settings. I still practice it regularly.

The meditation practice that I'm going to introduce you to in a few pages—or any meditation practice, for that matter—is not so difficult that only a certain kind of person can master it. You'll be able to do it, and I truly believe you're going to embrace it once you experience the payoffs. But I don't want to give you the false impression that you have to be a "perfect" meditator (whatever that means!). One thing I want you to know, though, is that even though meditation is a big part of my life, I still find it challenging at times. Meditation definitely requires some discipline—it's not a piece of cake—and, like everything else, your practice will probably ebb and flow. At times I find it boring, at other times absolutely enlightening. Sometimes I will go through periods when I do it every day, but I've also gone months without sitting on a meditation cushion. So go into it with acceptance. Don't feel you have to have the rigor of a sage sitting on a mountaintop. Just be you, and it will come.

STAY HEALTHIER, SMARTER—EVEN YOUNGER!— THROUGH MEDITATION

Meditation boosts vitality in so many ways, not the least by improving your health. It's well established, for instance, that meditation can lower blood pressure and heart rate, boost immunity (meditation has even been shown to reduce the incidence, severity, and duration of colds and flu), and reduce the production of the stress hormone cortisol. Meditators with arthritis, bad backs, and other maladies experience less pain than nonmeditators. Think of how much more alive chronic pain sufferers feel when they get some relief—all the vitality they once had comes rushing back in.

Research has shown meditation can do much, much more, but I won't overwhelm you with all the studies showing its health benefits. Instead, here are just three interesting ones that give you an idea of how little it takes to get some big improvements in your well-being. All three studies were conducted at the University of California, Los Angeles, one of the institutions at the forefront of meditation research.

Meditation can reduce inflammation—and loneliness.

Inflammation is associated with several different diseases, including heart disease and cancer. Loneliness is also linked to health maladies such as high blood pressure, depression, and eroded cognitive functioning. Could meditation have an effect on both inflammation and loneliness? Turns out it could. A 2012 study assigned forty adults ages fifty-five to eighty-five to either a mindfulness meditation group or a control group that did not meditate. After eight weeks of daily thirty-minute group sessions, the meditators reported less loneliness and, amazingly, showed a reduction in the expression of pro-inflammatory genes. Just more evidence that we aren't wholly at the mercy of the DNA we're dealt—the choices you make in life count, too.

Meditation can help fight depression—and aging.

Being a caregiver for someone with dementia is a very challenging job, so you might imagine that caregivers are the perfect test subjects for a study on the soothing benefits of meditation. In the 2013 study, UCLA researchers attempted to see if meditation could offer some stress relief by enlisting thirty-nine caregivers to either meditate (they engaged in a type of meditation called Kirtan Kriya) or listen to relaxing music for twelve minutes per day over the course of eight weeks. When the study was over, the meditation group had significantly lower levels of depressive symptoms, greater improvement in mental health, and a boost in their cognitive function as compared with the music listeners. The researchers also looked at biological signs of aging and found that the meditators had a 43 percent improvement in enzymes that keep cells young. Nice bonus, don't you think?

Meditation can also keep the brain young.

Staying mentally, not just physically, young is definitely a part of vitality, and here, too, meditation can help. In UCLA's Laboratory of Neuro Imaging, researchers first found that longtime meditators had more gray matter than control subjects, one reason meditators may be able to regulate their emotions under stress. Then, in a 2011 follow-up study, they discovered that meditators who had been practicing anywhere from five to forty-six years (they were devotees of various forms of meditation) had stronger connections between the regions of their brains and showed less age-related atrophy.

THE MINDFUL WAY

I consider meditation a *spiritual* practice, but not a religious one. Whatever your beliefs, meditation can connect you with the divine within you, or if that's too godly sounding for you, let's just say it connects you to the very nature of your being. At the same time, meditation is very humanizing. As David DeSteno, PhD, a psychologist at Northeastern University in Boston, has put it, "Meditation helps dissolve the artificial social distinctions—ethnicity, religion, ideology to name some—that tend to divide people." It may sound like a lot of heavy lifting for a practice that needn't take up much more than twenty minutes of your time per day, but meditation has an uncanny ability to bring people together instead of pulling them apart.

There are many different types of meditations, some of which are complex and others that are fairly simple. I have studied and taught a variety of them, but over the years my practice has shifted toward a simple yet powerful mindful meditation, and that is what I'd like to share with you here. Mindfulness helps you become an objective observer of your own life. Rather than encouraging you to block out certain thoughts and emotions, mindfulness teaches you to allow them to exist and to pass through you without judgment or criticism.

SEEDS OF WISDOM

Mindfulness is simply being aware of what is happening right now without wishing it were different; enjoying the pleasant without holding on when it changes (which it will); being with the unpleasant without fearing it will always be this way (which it won't).

—JAMES BARAZ, *mindfulness meditation teacher*

I've heard mindful meditation described as "unconditional friendli-ness to oneself." Isn't that delightful? Think of how freeing it would be to be as accepting of yourself as you probably are of your dearest friend. Mindfulness can put you on the path to being not only less judgmental and critical of yourself, but of other people as well.

What you learn from practicing mindful meditation also has great carryover. It is amazing how much more effective you become in dealing with life's inevitable stresses when you cultivate a practice of mindfulness and invite moments of awareness and stillness into your life. The mindfulness techniques you learn don't just exist for those twenty or so minutes you spend in meditation; they become a way of life. And when you bring your full attention to the present moment, as mindfulness teaches, life can radically shift. Your mood lifts, your body feels more relaxed, your mind becomes more open, you feel more confident and at peace, and your intuition comes "online." You can make this shift in a wink of an eye, too, just by consciously choosing to do so. And as your practice grows, you'll also find that you're less distracted, more adventurous, more exuberant, and, *ta-da*, more vital!

Here's a brief snapshot of what you do during a mindful medita-tion (I'll give you the step-by-step details shortly). You sit in a quiet place and focus on your breathing. As you do this, you let thoughts, feelings, and sensations gently move through your consciousness. You observe what comes up, viewing it with compassionate detach-ment without overanalysis or judgment, and always bring your atten-tion back to the present moment. During a mindful meditation, you become self-aware—which is very different from being self-involved or self-centered. Instead, it's becoming a conscious and objective observer of what *is*. You become very friendly with the present moment.

This is an abbreviated description, but that is the essence of what you will experience when practicing mindful meditation. Perhaps it seems like a bit of a leap from practicing this simple exercise to being able to go out into the world and focus better, handle stress with greater composure, control your impulses better, and begin taking responsibility for occurrences in your life that you might once have blamed on others. Yet every minute you spend in mindful meditation trains your brain to be present; it makes a moment-to-moment awareness second nature, so you not only experience life more fully, you can hear what your body, mind, and soul have to say. That last bit is no small thing. How much of your day is spent operating on autopilot, reacting in a rote manner to whatever arises? Mindfulness teaches you to act less out of habit and more in alignment with your true self.

THE DIFFERENCE BETWEEN MINDFULNESS AND RELAXATION

"It is important to note that [mindful meditation] is not the same as relaxation. While meditative practice may induce an integrated set of physiological changes (e.g., lowered heart, breathing, and metabolic rates), the practice of MM is an active and intentional state of awareness whose purpose is not, necessarily, to induce a state of relaxation. Unlike relaxation training, MM teaches individuals to attenuate prolonged reactivity to negative stimuli, whereas relaxation training encourages distraction and sleep may not be considered as an unwelcomed outcome during practice."

—FROM *PSYCHOLOGY RESEARCH AND BEHAVIOR MANAGEMENT*, 2012

MEDITATION AND THE MEANINGFUL, PURPOSEFUL LIFE

What do most people wish for every time they throw a coin in a fountain? I don't know for sure, but I bet at least half of them wish for some kind of improvement in their relationships or careers or in the lives of others they care about (the other half probably wish for the latest iPhone). Perhaps they wish for world peace. Even an NBA player (Ron Artest) changed his name to Metta World Peace in an effort to be inspirational (*metta* is a Sanskrit word for loving-kindness, friendliness, and benevolence). Fundamentally, I believe we all want the world to be a better place, but in the day-to-day shuffle of our own lives, compassion and kindness can get shoved under the rug. Yet is it really possible to have a truly meaningful and purposeful life without them? We derive meaning and purpose not only from what we take in from the world but from what we give out—and compassion and kindness are our most vital exports.

Because meditation is often billed as a way to reduce stress and induce relaxation—important aspects of it, for sure—it can seem like a purely self-centered exercise. Yet research shows that meditation can have an impact that reaches above and beyond the individual, actually helping to make the world a kinder and more compassionate place. How could you not feel more vital and alive when you know you're doing your part to promote world peace (or at least greater civility)?!

Okay, meditation may not be solving all the problems in the Middle East, but it really can help you make more of a positive contribution to society. Consider a study that came out of David DeSteno's Social Emotions lab at Northeastern University. The researchers under DeSteno's watch recruited thirty-nine people to undergo an eight-week meditation workshop. Nineteen of the people were told they were on the waiting list for the workshop, while the remaining twenty began taking part in weekly classes and using guided recordings to help them meditate at home. Ten of them also had discussions about compassion and suffering during the workshop.

After the eight weeks were up, the researchers invited the meditators as well as those on the waiting list to their lab, telling them they were going to participate in an experiment examining memory and other cognitive abilities. But that was just a ruse. Instead, the researchers wanted to see what would happen when the meditators and nonmeditators were confronted with a situation that tested their reaction to someone else's suffering. So they set up this situation: When the study participant walked into the waiting room of the lab, there was only one available chair for him or her to sit in; the other two chairs in the room were occupied. After a time, a woman on crutches with a broken foot entered the room and sighed in pain, in obvious discomfort as she leaned against the wall. The other people in the waiting room, who were plants, ignored the injured woman. The question, then, was, would the study participant act compassionately, especially in the face of the others' indifferent behavior?

You would think that everyone would be quick to offer a seat at the sound of that sigh, but that's not what happened. Only 16 percent of the nonmeditators gave up their seats; when it came to the meditators, the display of compassion was much higher—50 percent. The researchers concluded that something important had happened during the meditation sessions that led to greater humanity among the meditators. After the study was complete, DeSteno noted that meditation helps enhance awareness, which may have simply made the meditators pay more attention to what was happening in the waiting room than the nonmeditators. But his favored explanation (and mine) was that the compassionate response of the meditators "derives from a different aspect of meditation: its ability to foster a view that all beings are interconnected."

SEEDS OF WISDOM

The present moment is filled with joy and happiness. If you are attentive, you will see it.

—THICH NHAT HANH, *Vietnamese Buddhist monk*

MINDFULNESS HITS THE BIG TIME

For some, there still hovers an image around meditation of tie-dye and beads and guys with scraggly beards and drawstring pants sitting cross-legged in rooms smoky with incense. Oh sure, there still may be some of that (the '60s and '70s are experiencing a revival!), but for the most part, that is not the scene these days. Meditation, and particularly mindfulness, is appearing in the most modern and sophisticated of arenas, including universities, tech firms, corporations, and even a law school.

Academia has actually been onto mindfulness for a while. One of the early mainstream proponents of mindfulness meditation, Jon Kabat-Zinn, PhD , founded the Center for Mindfulness in Medicine, Health Care, and Society at the prestigious University of Massachusetts Medical School in 1979. Ellen J. Langer, PhD, a professor of psychology, has been studying mindfulness (without the meditation component) for over thirty years at Harvard. She has authored more than two hundred research mindfulness-related papers. Many universities, from University of California at San Diego to the University of Virginia to the University of Missouri, have mindfulness centers or programs.

More recently, corporations like Google and General Mills have instituted mindfulness programs. Google's mindfulness classes, called Search Inside Yourself, focus on attention training, self-knowledge and self-mastery, and the creation of useful mental habits. A General Mills lawyer started mindfulness training at the company, then went on to found an institute that introduces executives to the practice. Meditation techniques are also now being taught at some business schools like the Drucker School of Management at Claremont Graduate University outside Los Angeles, and in executive MBA programs such as those at Harvard University and the University of Michigan's Ross School of Business. (How appropriate that MBA stands for mind-body awareness, too.) Lawyers are getting in on it as well: UC Berkeley's School of Law recently announced the creation of the Berkeley Initiative for Mindfulness in Law, founded to "integrate the insights of meditation" into the work of students and faculty with the goal of making the legal system more just and compassionate.

Some people are a little skeptical about the intersection of true mindfulness and business, law, and other industries not particularly known for benevolence. But I'm all for it! If the captains of industry and justice have a more compassionate, humanistic outlook on life, the trickle-down will change the world for the better.

HOW TO MEDITATE

Mindfulness meditation is a bit like exercise: sometimes it's best to ease into it and build up your "muscles" as you go. First, set aside a time of day when you won't be interrupted. Next, choose an appropriate place (quiet helps with focus, but my first meditation classes were accompanied by the loud sound of a gardener's gas-powered leaf blower; it actually helped me develop a better ability not to be sidetracked by distractions!). It can sometimes be useful to meditate in a group or to take meditation classes. You might expect a group setting to be distracting, but it can help you to push yourself a bit further and more easily access a higher state of consciousness, especially with a group of trained meditators. I don't suggest becoming dependent on any group or teacher. A good teacher is one whose ultimate aim is not to have you become a follower, but rather to help you to become your own "guru."

I suggest that you begin by practicing the following set of meditation steps ten to fifteen minutes a day, working your way up, ideally, to a daily routine of anywhere from thirty to forty-five minutes. Set a timer if you like. Ready? Okay, here are your seven basic steps for meditation.

1. You can choose to sit on a cushion or pillow in a cross-legged position. OR if it's more comfortable for you, you can sit on a simple chair. Keep your spine straight, and allow your shoulders to soften and drop. Let your hands gently rest in your lap or place them with palms up or down on your knees.

2. Close your eyes, take a deep breath, and exhale fully, consciously releasing any tension you're holding in your body. Now take a scan of your body, moving from part to part, and releasing tension as you go, starting at your feet, moving to your calves, then thighs, hips, abdomen, back, shoulders, neck, and working up and relaxing the muscles in your jaw and the muscles behind your eyes.

3. Take another deep breath, and as you exhale, set aside any thoughts of things you have to do or emotions you're holding on to. The important things will be waiting for you at the end of your practice.

4. Bring your attention to the natural flow of your breath. With each inhale, allow yourself to become more comfortable and at ease. Inevitably you will be distracted by thoughts, feelings, noises, and sensations in your body (I'm all for scratching an itch if you need to). Don't push them away. Experience them, observe them, let them run their course, and keep your focus on your breathing. If you find yourself stuck in a

SEEDS OF WISDOM

Meditation is not a way of making your mind quiet. It's a way of entering into the quiet that's already there— buried under the 50,000 thoughts the average person thinks every day.

—DEEPAK CHOPRA, *physician and author*

particular thought or feeling, sometimes shifting a little on your cushion or chair and sitting up a little straighter can help you release it.

5. At this point, it sometimes helps to introduce a seed thought. A seed thought is an intention that you set toward the beginning of your meditation that focuses your energy. The thought can center around a specific quality, action, attitude, or state of being that you would like to more fully embody. You silently state it to yourself, then let it go, trusting that your intention has been made. It's not a mantra—a chant that you repeat over and over again—which can be helpful but tends to busy the mind, blocking out all the things you might otherwise be aware of, not what we're going for here; a seed thought can be anything you want but tends to work well when it's a positive statement about your being. An appropriate *Chia Vitality* seed thought might be *I stand receptive to a life filled with vitality, gratitude, and wholeness.* (It can be beneficial to work with the same seed thought for a week or more at a time, but it's not necessary.) Now allow the breath to find its own rhythm as you allow the seed thought to resonate throughout your being.

6. At some point, your seed thought will fall away and you will feel yourself move into a place of stillness. (If you become distracted—which you will—come back again to an awareness of the breath.) Try to sit in that stillness for as long as you can. This is the silent sound of your soul.

7. After the time is up or you feel complete, bring your awareness back to your breath. I like to end my meditation with an audible *Om*, or a silent *Om* if I am in a public place. When you feel ready, open your eyes. Place your hands together in prayer at your chest and bow your head. *Namaste* ("The soul within me honors the soul within you"). As you continue through your day, carry your seed thought with you.

Remember that meditation is an opportunity to cultivate more kindness and compassion, not an opportunity to judge yourself.

Meditation can be difficult and although it cultivates the higher aspects of yourself, it can also stir up the self-judging and critical parts, too. Be kind and hold an attitude of kindness and forgiveness.

MORNING AND EVENING MEDITATIONS

Even when life gets so busy that I don't take time out for any formal meditation, I begin and end the day with these two mini meditations. They're super simple and can help you stay in spiritual alignment and cope with days that swirl fast and furiously around you.

On waking:

Identify yourself as a soul—that is, an eternal, whole, and beautiful being that is part of the One Life—the interconnectedness of all living things. Dedicate yourself in service to the soul of humanity, the collective divinity of us all, and to the soul of the planet. Now set your intention for the day. This is not your practical to-do list, but your spiritual objectives. A few examples: *May I see the beauty in all things today and be filled with vitality and gratitude.* Or perhaps, *May I be filled with compassion and kindness for myself and others.* Or, *I trust in the Universe to help me be my highest and best self.*

Before going to sleep:

Identify as a soul once again and take a few minutes to review the day. I am a big fan of gratitude journals (the paper or computer-generated kind), but you can also "write" in your mental gratitude journal. Record what you're grateful for that happened during the day. It doesn't have to be big stuff; in fact, the little things that we experience each day that we are now more mindful of can bring such delight! Send out love and blessings to humanity and the planet, then allow yourself to drift off to sleep, trusting that you are connected to the One Life.

EVERYDAY MINDFULNESS

Everyday meditations can help you become fully present—life doesn't just pass you by . . . you really feel it! Your attitude toward your environment and its beautiful bounty (including your own body, emotions, and mind) becomes one of deep appreciation and gratitude. And these small meditations can be practiced in so many different ways. You can do them while you're washing the dishes (feel your hands in the water, the warmth of its temperature, and the movement of your fingers as you move the sponge, and so on), while cooking, while making the bed, while walking your dog—anything really.

In particular, being out in nature can be a great access point to mindfulness. For me, it's proven to be the ultimate mindfulness teacher. After a rough patch in my life, when I had aligned myself with a group that I thought was doing good in the world, only to find out they weren't very scrupulous, it was the practice of mindfulness through nature that helped bring me back into alignment with my soul. I had just left this painful situation and moved to our small farm in rural San Diego County. I sat under the avocado trees for hours on end, day after day, deeply appreciating the old trees, the soaring hawks, and the occasional roadrunner and coyote. I earnestly practiced mindfulness, allowing the restorative energy of forgiveness and gratitude to work its magic. It was after this deep dive into mindfulness that Mamma Chia was born—yet another reminder that what

SEEDS OF WISDOM

Don't ask what the world needs. Ask what makes you come alive, and go do it. Because what the world needs is people who have come alive.

-HOWARD THURMAN, *author, philosopher, and civil rights leader* may first appear and feel like our darkest moments can also prove to be one of our greatest opportunities. You just need to take the time to fully *be* present in the moment.

Trust me on this, the present moment is the easiest exit point out of pain and into greater acceptance, enthusiasm, and JOY. It holds all we need. When we are holding on to the old stories of our past and allowing them to define us, or when we are fearful of making mistakes in the future, or thinking that we are "not enough," then pain is guaranteed to ensue. But being open to whatever arises and trusting yourself to have the wisdom (not perfection!) to meet it head-on is living vitality with a capital *V.* It does take practice, but here's some good news: it doesn't need to take years to get there!

EVEN EATING CAN BE A MEDITATION

Mindfulness can make the mundane magical! Even eating a rice cracker with almond butter sprinkled with chia seeds can be a sacred and fully enchanting experience. Here's how to turn that simple act from a mechanical exercise into a meditation. As you prepare the cracker, bring your awareness to what your hands are doing. Feel the knife in your hand as you spread the almond butter and notice its aroma. When you bite into the cracker, be aware of its crackle and the differing sensations of the smooth almond butter and crunchy chia seeds in your mouth. Chew slowly so you really taste the food. Relish each bite. It doesn't have to even be this complicated. For instance, I love eating with chopsticks because it helps me to slow down and be more mindful (which as a bonus helps me avoid overeating as well).

7

·······

EXPANDING YOUR WORLD

Expanding your world may seem to have nothing to do with getting more chia into your diet—or the other parts of this 30-day program—but let me explain how, in fact, they're all intimately related. If you're feeling physically, emotionally, mentally, and spiritually depleted, vulnerable, and unsure of yourself, your inclination will be to pull inward. When you're down, becoming an engaged member of society can seem way too challenging. It's even hard to drag yourself to a cocktail party (and those are supposed to be fun). That's where the other spokes in this vitality wheel—the chia-based diet, the yoga, the meditation—come in. These things all shake you awake, opening your eyes and heart to the wider world out there. It seems to me that that can't help but boost your desire to participate and belong. And no doubt about it, becoming an active citizen of the world is a whole lot easier when you're feeling energetic and strong.

Once you begin venturing out, I think you'll also find that trying something new and meeting new people will only enhance your vitality. It's easy to get into a rut, doing the same things day after day. You may not feel noticeably bored, yet if you stop and think about it, life may have become rather dull! Connecting with community, becoming engaged in causes and pursuits that excite you, having new experiences—stretching yourself, in other words—can rouse your spirit in ways you didn't even realize you needed. It's like adding fuel to the vitality fire. When everything comes together, you're going to have one meaningful, purposeful, joyful life!

Starting any new business requires putting in some long, lonely hours, and I had plenty of those in the early days of Mamma Chia. But starting a *chia* business also had the wonderful dividend of connecting me to a whole new world of like-minded people and organizations. For all those lonesome hours I spent, I got paid back with the warmth and support of other people and an amazing sense of belonging. That experience cemented something for me that I've long believed: We are all part of a bigger whole. Connecting with others, being part of a community—any kind of community—doing service for and with others gives our lives more meaning and is so incredibly stimulating. Talk about a vitality boost! Ironically, one of the best ways to improve our inner lives is to look and move outward.

Before I get ahead of myself, I want to disabuse you of the notion that to get the vitality-enhancing benefits of community and service, you must be a live wire with a calendar-bursting social life or a volunteering schedule that rivals Mother Teresa's. Vital people aren't necessarily the life of the party or the people with the most friends on Facebook or the ladies that run a soup kitchen—although they can be. Vitality, remember, is the pursuit of mental vigor, growth, meaning, and purpose. When I talk about social connections and expanding your world, what I'm talking about is having a feeling of belonging as well as being part of something beyond yourself and your immediate circle. It's possible to attain all of these things whether you are or aren't an extrovert.

SEEDS OF WISDOM

I know there is strength in the differences between us.
I know there is comfort, where we overlap.

—Ani DiFranco, *singer/songwriter*

To some degree, all of us, whether shy or outgoing, are social crea-tures. We need to feel deeply connected to survive and especially to thrive. And research confirms just how much belonging feeds our bodies and souls. A sense of community, for instance, has been associ-ated with living longer, while loneliness has been linked with lower levels of immunity, inflammation, high blood pressure, and increased risk of cardiovascular disease and stroke. Being disconnected can make you feel more tired and even make you age faster. One study found loneliness has the same impact on your health as smoking fif-teen cigarettes a day! And, of course, you don't have to just be "alone" to feel lonely (anyone who's ever been trapped in a bad relationship knows that). Feeling detached or left out can make you feel nearly as lonely as living in isolation. And it's virtually impossible to have good health and well-being without connecting with others, soul-to-soul.

You undoubtedly live a busy life—who doesn't these days?—and that can make it seem as though there's no room for anything else. But in the spirit of seeking renewal through this 30-day program, I encourage you to do a little soul-searching. How connected to your community do you feel? Is there more you can do to enhance both your own life and the life of others? I bet the answer is yes!

WHAT CREATES COMMUNITY?

There are many different definitions of community, and some people place more emphasis on certain aspects than others. To me, having a sense of community is feeling a shared emotional, intellectual, and/or spiritual connection with others as well as a shared desire for the greater good. Community is a "place" where you can safely express your true self and get the support and opportunity you need to pursue your soul's purpose. One of the biggest motivators of human life is knowing that you're understood, heard, and appreciated. Community allows that to happen. Be on the lookout, though, for what I think of as false communities. Those are places where you must conform

SEEDS OF WISDOM

. . . .

We are healthy only to the extent that our ideas are humane.

—KURT VONNEGUT, *author*

to others' ideas, or where everyone must share *all* the same beliefs. Healthy and vibrant communities, on the other hand, allow you to share similarities while accepting (and even encouraging) the differences among you.

It's our good fortune to live in an age where we can even be part of virtual communities. It's a gift, too, to be able to so easily connect with friends and family who live far away and to connect with new people. And many romantic relationships are forged online these days. Still, technology can also give us ways to isolate ourselves from physical human contact, and nothing can replace eye contact or a big hug. It seems more important than ever, then, to make a conscious effort to be part of not just virtual communities, but real, living, breathing ones. And I think you can see a little bit of a backlash and a reaching out as people realize there's no substitute for human contact. I don't believe it's any accident that one of the biggest trends in restaurants is the communal table. Love them or hate them, they indicate a desire for connection and shared interests (and maybe even a shared bite or two!). Many cities are also finding ways to get more people to congregate in shared spaces, even if it's just a shopping mall with space for hanging out.

If you think about it, you may already be tangentially part of a community, but haven't reached out to any of the other "members." It could be the group of people who go to the same yoga studio as you. It could be the parents in your child's school. It could be a community related to your profession. Becoming a more active part of a community involves some risk; you have to allow yourself to be vulnerable and, if the connections don't work out as you hoped, resilient, too (the meditation in the previous chapter can help with this). When I moved to a new town, a friend I met in yoga told me she was in a great book club. I asked if she thought I might be able to join, and she said, "Oh no, we've been a group for ten years." I got it; they had something special going and probably didn't want to have to initiate someone new. Still, I was hurt. But I also consciously decided to keep my heart open and get back on the proverbial horse a short time later.

As I mentioned before, my start-up business put me in the path of a whole new crowd of people, who I discovered were like kindred spirits; it just took reaching out (as I said, getting back up on the horse) to engage with them. Before I launched Mamma Chia, I became a founding member of Slow Money, a nonprofit organization and movement that guides investment in small and local food enterprises. When I first read the Slow Money principles, I knew I needed to be a part of this movement. I didn't know exactly what that meant or what that would look like—I don't know if any of us did back then—but I did know that I needed to be at their Inaugural National Gathering in Santa Fe, New Mexico, back in 2009. And thank God I listened to myself and went. It turned out to be one of the most defining moments of my life—for me personally and, later, for Mamma Chia as well. The relationships that have been born and cultivated in this community are some of the most beautiful and enriching in my life. And I am delighted to say that there are now local Slow Money chapters across the country that are helping to build communities and support the local food movement.

Another incredible community I am a member of is the Social Venture Network, an organization that supports and inspires the building of a just and sustainable economy. SVN is filled with engaging and conscious souls who want to make a difference in the world. And they definitely know how to throw a good party—always a plus! Even though SVN is technically a professional group, belonging has changed my life in a deeply personal way, offering incredible support and rewarding friendships. Mamma Chia is also a member of several

SEEDS OF WISDOM

Community is a sign that love is possible in a materialistic world where people so often either ignore or fight each other. It is a sign that we don't need a lot of money to be happy—in fact, the opposite.

—JEAN VANIER, *philosopher, theologian, humanitarian*

incredibly dynamic communities that seed my soul, such as 1% for the Planet, a global movement of companies donating at least 1% of their annual sales to environmental organizations, and the B Corporation. Certified B corporations, like Mamma Chia, are businesses committed to serving the greater good that meet rigorous standards of social and environmental performance, accountability, and transparency. These kinds of groups are good for the soul of humanity and the soul of the planet!

The reason I bring up these organizations is to show you there are many different kinds of communities out there that likely reflect your values. You needn't belong to just one type of community (and I use the word *belong* informally, not necessarily in a dues-paying-member kind of way). What's more, no single community has to define your life or even be your main source of activity. These various communities, compartmentalized though they may be, can still be nurturing. Maybe it's the friends at the gym you've been going to for years, whom you never see outside the locker room but who've nonetheless seen you through some of your darkest times. Maybe it's your colleagues at work or the people in your wine club or the guys who eat breakfast at the same diner as you every morning. Community is everywhere if you're looking for it. Here are just a few places you might find it.

Nine Ways to Enlarge Your Circle

1. Join a community garden. Depending on where you live, this might not be a year-round option, but once spring hits, get your spade and seeds ready! Some community gardens are shared plots, while others allow you to have your own individual plot. Either way, they not only help cultivate interaction with like-minded garden lovers, they allow you to cultivate healthy food and flowers as well as beautify your neighborhood. The American Community Garden Association (communitygarden.org) can help you find a growing place near you.

2. Hang out at the dog park. A Canadian study found that people who walk their dogs four times or more a week have a more heightened sense of community than people who don't own a dog. It also helped them get in 150 minutes of walking a week, proving that dog walking is good for your health and your spirit. It may also enhance your sense of community if you walk your dog over to a communal dog park. Tight-knit communities (and probably a few romances) are known to blossom among animal lovers who get to know one another while their pooches play. Don't have a dog? Borrow one; your friend or family member will be grateful (and so will your furry friend).

3. Regularly attend a yoga or other fitness class. Bonds among devotees of a particular class tend to form over time, so consider finding a class you love and stick to it. The nice thing about exercise-related classes is that they are generally continuous; they don't end after a semester or session, so you can take your time getting to know the other participants. Sometimes it may take months (even years) for connections to gel, but they can be solid once they do.

4. Knit one, purl two. If you like to knit, or would like to learn, consider joining a knitting circle, often found at knit stores or even in people's homes. A website called stitchnbitch.org can help you find a group in your area, no matter where you live—it has links to groups all over the world! It's also got tips on how to start your own knitting circle.

5. *Meet up for shared pursuits.* Back in chapter 5, I mentioned meetup.com, a site for hooking up people who have mutual passions. It's not only a great resource for exercisers, it can open the door to all kinds of people-populated activities, ranging from foodie crawls to music lover clubs to writers' groups and cultural salons. You can find knitting groups here, too (see #4). Be brave while being careful, of course.

6. *Take the idea of community literally.* Get involved in your neighborhood or city. Join groups that help keep your area safe, clean, vital, and beautiful. This is a great opportunity to not only help get things done where you live but find ways to truly love thy neighbor.

7. *Look for farm-to-table events.* These get-togethers, meals that allow you to sample local food and wine with people on the same wavelength, are becoming increasingly popular around the country. Sometimes they meet in restaurants, sometimes on farms or at wineries. It's a great introduction to companions who care about what they eat as well as the earth that supplies this wonderful bounty.

8. *Participate in online communities.* As I've mentioned before, I believe there's no substitute for in-person interaction. Eye contact, the human touch, hugs!—nothing can replace these. That said, I also think that online social networking does represent a new kind of shared mind that taps into the collective consciousness of our society. How amazing is it that we can now connect to millions of people all over the world? It definitely enhances life. Online communities can move mountains. As an entrée to one that moves *you*, look for blogs on topics you care about, join professional listservs, check out Facebook activity, or just simply search around in Google. Observe until you find a group that interests you, then point your cursor and jump in.

9. *Walk this way.* Walking groups are one of the best ways to get a feeling of community. First of all, there are hundreds of them, and it's easy to start your own; just call up friends, have them call their friends, and so on. Secondly, there's a sort of intimacy that develops as you walk that can open your soul. Maybe it's the feel-good effect of the exercise (and the pace of a fitness activity that allows you to still talk), but walkers often grow close. Stick with it and before you know it, magic will happen.

SERVING EVERYBODY'S NEEDS

By now it may be cliché, but I always loved that bumper sticker slogan PRACTICE RANDOM ACTS OF KINDNESS. Everyday kindnesses are often taken for granted; however, they play a considerable roll in lifting the overall mood of a community. The political satirist P. J. O'Rourke has said "Everybody wants to save the Earth; nobody wants to help Mom do the dishes." Besides being funny, I think it points out that the small touches of benevolence often get pushed aside in favor of the grander gestures. But the small things are no less significant. And, let's be honest, being kind and helpful makes you feel really good about yourself. You feel vital because you *are* vital. It can be so simple, too.

Smiling is the perfect example. Have you ever heard of what psychologists call "emotional contagion"? Cells in your brain record the emotional expressions of other people, then send a message to your muscles to follow suit. If someone is smiling at you, the muscles around your mouth and eyes will contract, and you will smile, too. You catch smiling just like a bug! But there is more than mere mimicry involved. You also get a wave of the happy emotions that smiling represents. It changes your internal state as well as your external state. So you can see why the simple act of smiling at someone is a gift, especially since smiling activates feel-good chemicals in the body that deflect stress and can even lower heart rate and blood pressure.

If you can take on bigger acts of generosity, I urge you to give yourself the gift of helping another person. At one of the lower points of my illness, I decided that the best thing I could do would be to help someone else. There weren't a lot of ways I could be of service in those days, but driving, most times, was something I could do. The job I volunteered for was driving late-stage AIDS patients to their doctors' appointments. You probably know what I'm going to say next: It was one of the most fulfilling experiences of my life.

Often when people know that they have a very limited time to live, their priorities become very clear. They don't waste their time and energy on nonessentials or petty things. The souls that I met on this journey deeply inspired me with their bravery and grace. I often witnessed acts of forgiveness that healed families and opened hearts to greater love and gratitude. It was a privilege and honor to be with them.

Another opportunity to serve presented itself when a new Alzheimer's center opened in our community. It didn't have a volunteer program at the time, but that didn't stop me from finding out how I could get involved. So I helped the center initiate a program to bring more love and connection to the residents. I led basic exercise classes, and my husband socialized the center's dogs and cat with the residents. Both experiences opened my heart and mind in ways I couldn't have foreseen. Service is almost always just as beneficial to the one doing the giving as it is to the one doing the receiving—if not more so. In fact, it provides one of the best opportunities available to feel vital and alive.

Perhaps that's because altruism, at least as I see it, is part of our basic nature. Even though it can be sublimated, pushed down by circumstance or because our lives get so crazy it's hard to see beyond our own noses, I think we all have the impulse to serve in some way. But we are more than our brothers' and sisters' keepers. We *are* our brothers and sisters. A tremendous and dynamic change happens when we break free of the illusions of separation. When we truly understand that everything—from the president of the United States to the tiniest ant to the trees and the stars—is interconnected, we become a very powerful and effective agent for good in the world. I think we all have the potential to become world servers and to live a life filled with vitality, meaning, and purpose.

World servers are those individuals who are consciously working toward the greatest good of all. They do not see themselves as special, better, or less than their fellow human beings. They have an understanding of the interconnectedness of all life. As you can see, my definition of world servers is all encompassing. It includes professions that by definition help other people or the planet. It includes people who give of their time, and perhaps money, to do good. But it also includes the person who smiles at you in the grocery checkout line and says hello to you as you pass by on the street. It's the person who holds the door for you, who motions you to go ahead at the stop sign or gives up a seat to you on the bus. World servers are found in every arena of human living and are not confined to any one group of people. Their service is practical, inclusive, and lovingly motivated. Some world servers are easily identified on the world stage—who doesn't think of Mother Teresa as a prominent example—but, more commonly, they are found quietly serving the common good through their families and local communities, thereby uplifting the consciousness of the whole.

By becoming world servers, we can live more effective and joy-filled lives while consciously co-creating a better world. You're probably already offering love, kindness, and service to the world in some way. Sometimes all you need to do to help someone is to be present, fully present, and just let that person *be*. Maybe, though, I've also now got you thinking about trying to contribute in a bigger or different way. Here are a few things that might help you get involved:

- **Set a reasonable goal.** Once you decide you'd like to get involved with a cause, zeal can set in and cause you to overcommit. Overcommitting can lead you to feel overwhelmed by the responsibility of the task at hand and usually leads you to end up quitting entirely rather than pulling back to a more modest commitment. I'm all for taking a deep dive into things—it's part of my own nature to do so—but here I urge you to take your time. Maybe start by reserving one day out of the month for volunteer work. That's such a modest goal that even the busiest of people can usually stick to it. If it feels right, you can then work up from there.

- **Narrow down the list.** There are no shortages of ways to get involved. The easiest way to find an opportunity is to go to the website of an organization you admire, then get in touch. There are also groups that are in business of matchmaking volunteers with volunteering opportunities. If you have an interest in, say, feeding the homeless, they can point you in the right direction. Volunteermatch.org is one; Volunteers of America (voa.org) is another.

- **Think about using the skills you already have.** Volunteering isn't all soup kitchens, building Habitat for Humanity bungalows, or beach cleanups (worthy though they are). Your professional skills or even personal proficiencies may be just what a nonprofit needs. Whether you have a knack for computer programming, communications, accounting, graphic design, or any one of a myriad of skills, there's likely a place for you. Check out Catchafire (catchafire.org), a group that matches professionals who want to do good with organizations that need their help.

SEEDS OF WISDOM

I slept and I dreamed that life is all joy. I woke and I saw that life is all service. I served and I saw that service is joy.

—KHALIL GIBRAN, *inspirational writer*

SEEDS OF KNOWLEDGE

THE ALTRUISM DIVIDEND

There's no doubt that being on the receiving end of love, kindness, and support is beneficial. Researchers have found all kinds of evidence that recipients have lower rates of disease and, on the flip side, that the loss of love can depress the immune system. But what about the altruistic givers? They benefit, too.

For one thing, people who volunteer live longer than people who don't. One 1999 study found that the health advantages of volunteering were even greater than those that came from exercising four times a week and nearly as great as those from quitting smoking. Isn't that amazing? It just goes to show how much our mind and spirit affect our bodies. What's even more amazing is how altruism influences emotions and state of mind. In 2008, a researcher at the London School of Economics named Francesca Borgonovi analyzed data on volunteering in the United States collected by the John F. Kennedy School of Government at Harvard University. She found that people who volunteer are happier than people who don't. (Altruism has also been linked to improved morale, better self-esteem, and less depression.) What the volunteering data also showed, though, was that while having little money was associated with unhappiness in people who *didn't* volunteer, volunteers were happy whether they were rich or poor. Pondering the results, Borgonovi posed the idea that volunteering might reinforce satisfaction for what one has rather than dissatisfaction for what one lacks.

How right she is! Even the smallest of things, like bringing a meal to a friend who is sick or helping an elderly person carry her groceries, makes you feel not only more satisfied with your own circumstances, but *grateful*. It truly gives meaning and purpose to life, and that's the best kind of vitality boost you can get.

MOVING OUT OF YOUR COMFORT ZONE

One thing I discovered when I started Mamma Chia is that if you keep an open mind and heart, you end up learning, growing, and assembling good people around you. At our company, we make a point of celebrating the diverse ideology among us. Democrat, Republican, Independent, Jewish, Christian, Buddhist, atheist—we're all here at Mamma Chia. This isn't a lecture on diversity, tolerance, and inclusiveness—our society is so polarized these days that there are plenty of people out there already doing the work of trying to bring us all back together. However, I did want to share my observation that expanding your world to include people who think differently than you do can be a joyful and even an eye-opening experience. In diversity there is beauty and strength—and that makes way for more vitality!

Inclusiveness gets a lot of lip service, but it's not practiced that often. It's easy—and at times I've been as guilty as anyone—to shut down and tune out ideas that don't appear to be in total alignment with our perceived notions of what's best. The fact is, many of us share core values; we just have different ideas of how to reach the same goals. Finding the middle ground—focusing on things that unite, not divide removes all the vitality-killing negativity from the equation. We all have challenges, triumphs, and disappointments in our lives; we are all interconnected souls. Remember that as you go through life, and you will feel lighter, more carefree, and endlessly vital.

SEEDS OF WISDOM

As you discover what strength you can draw from your community in this world from which it stands apart, look outward as well as inward. Build bridges instead of walls.

—SONIA SOTOMAYOR, *Supreme Court justice*

8

· · · · · ·

PUTTING IT ALL TOGETHER . . .
AND MAKING IT LAST

believe strongly that there's no one ideal way to live life—seemingly
odd words from someone who has just handed you a "prescription"
for a vitality-boosting mode of living. My intent has always been to
share with you the magic of chia and its many benefits, along with the
other life-enhancing elements that I (and lots of other people) have
found to work synergistically to bring more vitality, joy, and meaning
to one's life. Thirty days, I hope, will be just enough time to give you
a taste of how renewed, strong, energetic, and vibrant putting it all
together can make you feel.

After you've taken the leap of exposing yourself to new things for
30 days, you can begin making adjustments in the plan to make it fit
into your life. I fully expect that after the 30 days, you will take all
these elements, shuffle them around, and create your own personal
program. After all, you will have become not only a chia expert, but
adept at listening to the wisdom of your own body and soul. Hopefully, you'll also build on everything you sampled in the *Chia Vitality*
program, including all the tasty chia dishes, and be eager to spread the
chia love all around!

Ultimately, there are two factors that will help you turn the changes
you make during the *Chia Vitality* program into an ongoing part of
your life. The first is becoming aware of and accepting the present
moment, as well as grateful for all that you are experiencing. Simply
by virtue of revving you up and making your life more purposeful

151

and meaningful, the combination of chia, yoga, meditation, and service will give you the inspiration and tools you need to stay on course. You'll become a devotee simply because it feels so good! The second thing that will make these new habits last is knowing that you can attain vitality without being perfect. Letting go of the idea that you must do everything—and do everything flawlessly—is liberating. Remember, perfectionism is the enemy of vitality. So let go of trying to be perfect, and replace it with trying to be perfectly in the moment. What *Chia Vitality* does require is an open heart and an open mind and heaps of kindness and compassion for yourself and others. And heaps of chia, too!

Over the last few years, rarely a day goes by that someone doesn't reach out to me and share how chia has changed his or her life. Having experienced firsthand the power of these little seeds, I am deeply appreciative to have them in my life. All the omega-3s, protein, fiber, calcium, and other nutrients packed into their tiny interiors, their super-revitalizing effects, the way the seeds are so easily worked into every kind of dish—I don't know of another food that can boast so many great qualities and do so much for you.

It fills me with so much joy and gratitude to be following my soul's purpose and, at the same time, to be helping others to follow theirs. It is my hope that you, too, will experience better health, greater vibrancy, and a more meaningful and purposeful life. So it is with love and joy that I offer *Chia Vitality* to you. *Namaste.*

What follows is a *suggestion* of how you might put together all the pieces of this program. I say *suggestion,* because each of our lives is unique—what works for one person might not work for the next. You'll know just how much you can fit into your life and will follow suit. That said, if you think that meditating every day or doing yoga three times a week is too challenging, remember that it's only 30 days of your life. Try to shoot for the max. If you say to yourself, *Okay, I can do it; it's only for a brief time*, it will help you power through. And you might actually surprise yourself. I bet by the end of the 30 days you're not going to want to give up these healthy new habits!

30 DAYS OF *CHIA VITALITY*

These are just suggestions for how you might pace yourself over the next 30 days. Yoga is such a great way to start the day, but sometimes in the morning the pressure to get your day going can make finding the time more difficult, so feel free to make it an evening practice if mornings don't work for you. To shorten or lengthen your yoga practice, simply do fewer or more repetitions than called for in the sequence beginning on page 198. I find meditation to be most beneficial in the morning, to set the intention and tone of my day, but again, feel free to move it to the evening if it's a little bit easier then to calm your thoughts and ease into a meditative state. See what works best for you, then set your schedule accordingly. I've also added a seed thought to aid in your meditation practice each day. Also feel free to develop seed thoughts of your own that will support you on the path to greater vibrancy and a more meaningful and purposeful life.

Days 1–6
Preplan: The *Chia Vitality* Cleanse (optional)

Seed Thought: I quiet my mind and tune in to the innate wisdom of my body.

Practice 10 minutes of meditation each day, using this week's seed thought.

Enjoy foods from the meal plan.

Alternate between 15 minutes of yoga practice and mindful walking per day. Use the yoga practice on pages 198–214 to get started.

Bedtime Alignment: Align with your soul and acknowledge the innate wisdom of your body. Consciously send love, gratitude, and kindness out into the world. Be sure to include yourself.

Days 7–12

Seed Thought: I am open to a life of love, laughter, and vitality.

Practice at least 10 minutes of meditation per day using this week's seed thought. On day 12, try 20 minutes.

Enjoy foods from the meal plan.

Alternate between 20 minutes of yoga practice and mindful walking each day.

Bedtime Alignment: Align with your soul and feel your life being filled with love, laughter, and vitality. Consciously send love, gratitude, and kindness out into the world. Be sure to include yourself.

Days 13–18

Seed Thought: I greet the world and myself with kindness, compassion, and gratitude.

Practice at least 15 minutes of meditation per day using this week's seed thought.

Enjoy food from the meal plan. If you're having trouble keeping up, try some of the easy chia add-ins on page 52.

Alternate between 20 minutes of mindful walking and yoga practice each day.

Bedtime Alignment: Align with your soul and consciously send love, gratitude, and kindness out into the world. Be sure to include yourself.

Days 19–24

Seed Thought: I trust Life and know that all is working out for my highest good.

Practice 30 minutes of meditation at least 2 days this week
using this week's seed thought.

Enjoy foods from the meal plan. Try new recipes this week, or
remake your favorites from earlier in the program.

Elevate your physical activity by making time for 30 minutes
of mindful walking each day, and practicing 20 minutes of
yoga every other day.

*Bedtime Alignment: Align with your soul and know that all
is working out for your highest good. Consciously send
love, gratitude, and kindness out into the world. Be sure to
include yourself.*

Days 25–30

Seed Thought: Vitality and joy fills every cell of my Being.

Practice 30 minutes of meditation each day using this week's
seed thought.

Enjoy foods from the meal plan.

Engage your body with 30 minutes of mindful walking every
day, and practice 25 minutes of yoga every other day.

*Bedtime Alignment: Align with your soul and experience
vitality and joy dancing in every cell of your Being.
Consciously send love, gratitude, and kindness out into the
world. Be sure to include yourself.*

9

·······

NOW YOU'RE COOKING:

THE *CHIA VITALITY* RECIPES

D
o you remember how I talked about the benefits of synergy earlier in the book? You're about to experience it at its best. When
you sit down to eat these chia-centric dishes, you'll be getting
the nourishment you need to make you percolate with vigor and good
health. As you prepare them, you'll also be heightening your vitality
in another way: cooking is one of the best forms of mindful meditation there is. Just as in a sitting meditation, you have an opportunity
to be very focused and present as you cook. None of these recipes are
complicated or take long to make, but the time you do spend in the
kitchen will be time that heightens your spiritual and mental energy.
You're getting a double vitality boost here.

I hope these recipes will not only satisfy you but also inspire you
to think up new ways to use chia. If you're anything like I was when I
first discovered how easy it is to cook with the seeds, you'll start working chia or chia gel into almost everything. (Don't be surprised if you
get a few raised eyebrows when you begin tossing them into the sacro-
sanct holiday recipes your family has been eating for generations, but
stand your ground! They won't notice the taste, but they may notice
how good they feel.) There really is no end to the ways you can use
chia, so go forth and multiply your chia-based repertoire.

As I mentioned in chapter 4, I sometimes specify that a recipe
ingredient should be organic or non-GMO when I believe it's a particularly good idea. However, even when it's not stated, I recommend

choosing as many non-GMO, organic, or sustainably produced foods as possible. Of course, it's your choice, and you should do what's best for your budget and pantry.

Additionally, I recommend using PFOA-free pans. PFOA stands for perfluorooctanoatic acid, a chemical used to create nonstick surfaces, which may leach out into food; to be safe, use PFOA-free.

CHIA GEL

This handy little chia derivative has a Jell-O-like texture and allows you to thicken recipes while at the same time making their main ingredients go farther. For instance, when you add chia gel to a salad dressing, you don't have to use as much oil to get the amount you need to coat your lettuce leaves. The gel doesn't add any flavor; it just adds a nice body to recipes. And it's simple to make. Here's how:

Makes slightly more than 1 cup

Whisk together 1 cup of room-temperature purified water and 2 tablespoons of black or white chia seeds. Let stand for at least 20 minutes. Use immediately or store well covered in the refrigerator for up to 1 week. It's okay to double this recipe, if desired.

SEEDS OF WISDOM

Cooking demands attention, and above all, a respect for the gifts of the earth. It is a form of worship, a way of giving thanks.

—JUDITH B. JONES, *legendary editor of cookbooks*

BREAKFAST

. . . .

STEEL-CUT "SUPERFOOD" OATMEAL

If you are familiar with only rolled oats, I hope I inspire you to try steel-cut oats instead—they are particularly nutritious and, oh, so yummy. Nuttier and chewier than rolled oats, they take longer to cook but are worth the wait. You'll note that I advise buying gluten-free oats. Oats are naturally gluten free but are sometimes processed near grains that contain gluten, so you may want to seek out a packaged variety that is labeled gluten free. Since I am not overly gluten sensitive, I buy mine in the bulk section of my local natural foods store. This recipe also calls for cooking the oats in half juice, half water, which gives them a slight sweetness. For less sugar and fewer calories, use all water.

Makes three 1-cup servings

> *1½ cups 100% unsweetened organic apple juice*
> *1 teaspoon ground cinnamon*
> *½ teaspoon sea salt*
> *¼ teaspoon pure vanilla extract*
> *½ cup gluten-free steel-cut oats*
> *⅓ cup dried tart cherries or cranberries*
> *2 tablespoons black chia seeds*
> *3 tablespoons roasted and lightly salted pumpkin seeds*

1. In a medium saucepan over medium-high heat, bring the juice, cinnamon, salt, vanilla, and 1½ cups water just to a boil.

2. Stir in the oats, cherries, and chia seeds and return to a boil. Reduce heat to medium-low and simmer, uncovered, until cooked through, about 30 minutes, stirring occasionally.

3. Spoon the oatmeal into three cereal bowls, sprinkle with the pumpkin seeds, and serve while hot.

Per serving: 300 calories, 8 g total fat, 1 g saturated fat, 0 g trans fat, 410 mg sodium, 49 g total carbohydrate, 11 g dietary fiber, 18 g sugars, 9 g protein.

CHIA GRANOLA

The great thing about granola is that you can take a basic recipe and tweak it to your own tastes. Experiment with different sweeteners (honey works well), nuts and seeds (walnuts and sunflower seeds, for instance), as well as other types of dried fruit (such as chopped dried figs, dried cranberries, and dried tart cherries).

Makes fifteen ½-cup servings

> 6 cups gluten-free old-fashioned oats, such as Bob's Red Mill
>   Gluten-Free Old Fashioned Rolled Oats
> ½ cup extra-virgin olive oil
> ½ cup pure maple syrup, or more to taste
> 1 teaspoon ground cinnamon
> Pinch of sea salt
> 1 cup mixed nuts and seeds, such as unsalted chopped pecans,
>   sliced almonds, and pumpkin seeds
> ¼ cup black chia seeds
> ½ cup black seedless raisins

1. Preheat the oven to 300°F.
2. Place the oats in a large bowl. Add the olive oil, maple syrup, cinnamon, and salt, and toss to coat.
3. Transfer the mixture to two rimmed baking sheets. Bake for 10 minutes, stir, then bake for another 10 minutes. Stir in the nuts and seeds, including the chia seeds, and continue baking until the oat mixture is golden, about another 10 minutes.
4. Remove from the oven and stir in the raisins. Allow to cool, transfer to a lidded container, and store in a cool, dry place.

Per serving: 290 calories, 15 g total fat, 2 g saturated fat, 0 g trans fat, 0 mg cholesterol, 15 mg sodium 36 g total carbohydrate, 5 g dietary fiber, 11 g sugars, 6 g protein.

· ·

CALIFORNIA FRITTATA

This savory, fresh-tasting frittata incorporates Chia Gel (page 157) into the mix. Chia gel makes a great egg substitute on its own (see page 51 for details), so when you add it to a frittata, it's like adding a couple of additional eggs—but without the saturated fat. This frittata can be finished off one of two ways: on the stovetop, by placing a plate over the pan, or by slipping the pan (if it's ovenproof) under the broiler.

Makes four 1-wedge servings

>   4 large organic eggs
>   ⅓ cup Chia Gel (page 157)
>   ½ teaspoon sea salt, or to taste
>   2 teaspoons extra-virgin olive oil
>   1 large garlic clove, minced
>   1 (5-ounce) package fresh baby spinach (5 cups packed)
>   20 grape tomatoes, quartered
>   2 tablespoons finely chopped fresh basil + 4 small sprigs fresh basil,
>   for garnish
>   2 teaspoons fresh lemon juice
>   ½ Hass avocado, pitted, peeled, and sliced

1. Preheat the broiler (if using).

2. In a medium bowl, whisk together the eggs, chia gel, and ¼ teaspoon of the salt until combined. Set aside.

3. In a medium (10-inch, PFOA-free) nonstick skillet, heat the oil over medium-high heat. Add the garlic and sauté until fragrant, about 30 seconds. Add the spinach in batches, tossing with tongs until wilted, about 2 minutes. Add the tomatoes, chopped basil, lemon juice, and the remaining ¼ teaspoon salt and gently toss to combine. Cook about 1 minute and spread evenly across the skillet.

4. Pour the egg mixture over the spinach-tomato mixture. Shake the pan slightly to allow the egg mixture to fully settle. Cook until the eggs are fully set around the edges, about 5 minutes, tilting the

pan about halfway through the cooking process to let any uncooked egg on top run to the underside of the frittata. Cover, remove from the heat, and let stand until the eggs are completely set, about 3 minutes. (Alternatively, if skillet is ovenproof, place it under the broiler for 1 minute for the eggs to set.)

5. Slide the frittata onto a platter and slice into four wedges. Top with the avocado slices and the basil sprigs and serve.

Per serving: 150 calories, 10 g total fat, 2.5 g saturated fat, 0 g trans fat, 185 mg cholesterol, 420 mg sodium, 9 g total carbohydrate, 4 g dietary fiber 2 g sugars, 8 g protein.

. . . .

FRESH STRAWBERRY-CHIA SEED JAM

You don't even have to cook this jam—it's *that* easy—and the play between sweet and sour puts it very high on the deliciousness meter. If strawberries aren't in season, rather than buying a basket that's been shipped from thousands of miles away, I suggest buying your favorite low-sugar jam in a jar and combining it with Chia Gel (page 157)— about 2 tablespoons gel per half cup jam—or replacing the strawberries with another fruit that's in season.

Makes twenty 2-tablespoon servings

1 pound fresh organic strawberries, hulled and halved
¼ cup black chia seeds
3 tablespoons honey or agave nectar
2 teaspoons white balsamic vinegar or fresh lemon juice

1. In a food processor or blender, pulse the strawberries, chia seeds, honey, and vinegar until well combined, but not fully puréed.

2. Transfer to a bowl, cover, and chill for at least 4 hours. Store for up to 10 days in the refrigerator.

Per serving: 25 calories, 0.5 g total fat, 0 g saturated fat, 0 g trans fat, 0 mg cholesterol, 0 mg sodium, 5 g total carbohydrate, 1 g dietary fiber, 4 g sugars, 1 g protein.

. . . .

BLUEBERRY BUCKWHEAT PANCAKES

These pancakes are just as scrumptious with frozen blueberries as with fresh, so you can make them year-round. Maple syrup is key to their great taste, so use a real maple syrup, not a pancake syrup based on high-fructose corn syrup.

Makes four single 6- to 7-inch pancake servings

⅔ cup buckwheat flour
2 tablespoons milled (ground) chia seeds
1 teaspoon baking powder
¼ teaspoon sea salt
2 teaspoons cold unsalted organic butter, cut into tiny pieces
1 tablespoon honey or agave nectar
1 large organic egg
¾ cup plain unsweetened almond milk or other plant-based milk
½ teaspoon pure vanilla extract
1 cup fresh or thawed frozen blueberries
1 extra-small or ½ large banana, sliced crosswise or diced
¼ cup maple syrup, warmed

1. Preheat the oven to 200°F.

2. In a medium bowl, combine the flour, milled chia seeds, baking powder, salt, butter, and honey. Using a pastry blender or fork, mix until fine crumbs form.

3. In a large bowl, whisk together the egg, almond milk, and vanilla until well combined. Add the flour mixture and whisk again until thoroughly mixed. Let stand for 5 minutes. Stir ½ cup of the blueberries into the batter.

4. Lightly coat a large (PFOA-free) nonstick skillet or stick-resistant griddle with cooking spray and place over medium heat. Spoon the batter, about ½ cup per pancake, onto the hot surface and spread with the back of the spoon to flatten slightly, or by shaking the pan, to form a 6- to 7-inch pancake. Cook the pancakes in batches until

lightly browned, about 3 minutes on the first side and 2 minutes on the flip side. Transfer the pancakes after cooked to a heatproof platter. Keep warm in the oven until ready to serve

5. Sprinkle the pancakes with the banana, the remaining ½ cup of the blueberries, and serve with the maple syrup.

Per serving: 240 calories, 6 g total fat, 2 g saturated fat, O g trans fat, 50 mg cholesterol, 320 mg sodium, 41 g total carbohydrate, 6 g dietary fiber, 25 g sugars, 6 g protein.

LUNCH

· ·

MEDITERRANEAN TUNA SALAD

Chia gel lets you cut the mayo in this tuna salad by half! If you prefer chicken salad to tuna, simply replace the fish with an equal amount of shredded rotisserie chicken.

Makes four ½-cup servings

> 3 tablespoons Chia Gel (page 157)
> Juice and zest of 1 small lemon (2 tablespoons juice)
> 2 tablespoons mayonnaise, such as Follow Your Heart Organic
>   Vegenaise or Sir Kensington's Classic Mayonnaise (which is
>   non-GMO)
> ½ teaspoon sea salt, or to taste
> ¾ teaspoon freshly ground black pepper, or to taste
> 2 (5-ounce) cans water-packed sustainably caught albacore tuna with
>   no salt added, such as Wild Planet Wild Albacore Tuna, drained
>   and separated into chunks
> 1 medium stalk celery, finely diced
> ⅓ cup finely chopped red onion
> 6 pitted kalamata olives, thinly sliced (optional)
> 3 tablespoons chopped fresh flat-leaf parsley
> 2 tablespoons finely chopped fresh basil

1. In a medium bowl, stir together the chia gel, lemon juice and zest, mayonnaise, salt, and pepper until well combined.

2. Add the tuna, celery, onion, olives (if using), parsley, and basil and mix thoroughly. Cover and chill in the refrigerator until ready to serve.

3. Adjust seasonings and serve as is in a small bowl, as a sandwich filling, or in a hollowed-out tomato cup.

Per serving: 140 calories, 6 g total fat, 0.5 g saturated fat, 0 g trans fat, 30 mg cholesterol, 390 g sodium, 3 g total carbohydrate, 1 g dietary fiber, 1 g sugars, 17 g protein.

THAI TOFU PEANUT CHIA NOODLES

This is a great go-to dish when you're pressed for time. Buckwheat noodles cook up more rapidly than regular pasta, and since the recipe calls for prebaked tofu, you don't have to fool around with prepping your protein. Think ahead, and you can even make the sauce the day before, so all you've got to do is boil up the noodles, toss them with the rest of the ingredients, and sit down to a scrumptious chia meal.

Makes four rounded 1-cup servings

8 ounces dry 100% buckwheat soba noodles
¾ cup Thai Peanut-Chia Sauce (recipe follows)
6 ounces Asian-flavored baked organic tofu, cubed
2 cups thinly sliced unpeeled English or Persian cucumber or peeled
    and seeded regular cucumber
¼ cup roughly chopped fresh cilantro
4 lime wedges, for garnish

1. Boil the noodles according to package directions. Drain, rinse with cold water until cool, and drain well.

2. In a large bowl, toss together the noodles, peanut-chia sauce, tofu, cucumber, and cilantro to combine.

3. Transfer the noodle mixture to a serving bowl or individual bowls and serve at room temperature with the lime wedges on the side.

Per serving: 380 calories, 10 g total fat, 1.5 g saturated fat, 0 g trans fat, 910 mg sodium, 55 g total carbohydrate, 7 g dietary fiber, 7 g sugars, 19 g protein.

THAI PEANUT-CHIA SAUCE

Makes about 1½ cups

⅓ cup creamy no-added-sugar peanut butter
1 cup unsweetened freshly brewed green tea
3 tablespoons tamari soy sauce
Juice of 1 lime (2 tablespoons)
2 tablespoons black chia seeds
1 tablespoon honey or agave nectar
1 tablespoon freshly grated ginger
½ teaspoon hot pepper flakes, or to taste

In a small saucepan, stir together the peanut butter, tea, soy sauce, lime juice, chia seeds, honey, ginger, and hot pepper flakes until combined. Cook while stirring over medium heat until the sauce is slightly thickened and gently bubbling, about 8 minutes.

Transfer the sauce to a bowl and use immediately or store in a covered container in the refrigerator for up to 1 week. Gently warm the sauce before using, if necessary. Use with Thai Tofu Peanut Chia Noodles and/or as a sauce for grilled chicken skewers.

TROPICAL QUINOA AND KALE

Quinoa, kale, and chia—could there be a healthier trio? It just so happens that they also taste fantastic together, especially when accented with tropical coconut and pineapple flavors. Unless you're using baby kale (which is more tender and seems to be in markets more often these days), you'll need to remove the thick center stems from the kale leaves. An easy way to do it is to lay the leaf flat on a surface, place a knife the length of the leaf right up against the stem, then, holding the bottom of the stem, lift upward—the leaf will tear away from the spine. Repeat on the other side.

Makes four 1⅓-cup servings

> 1 13.5-ounce can organic light coconut milk, such as Native Forest
>   Organic Light Coconut Milk
> 1 cup quinoa, rinsed and drained
> 1½ tablespoons freshly grated ginger
> 1 tablespoon black chia seeds
> 1 large garlic clove, minced
> 10 ounces chopped fresh kale, thick stems removed
> ½ cup finely diced fresh pineapple, drained
> Juice of ½ lime (1 tablespoon)
> 1 teaspoon tamari soy sauce
> ¾ teaspoon sea salt, or to taste

1. In a large saucepan or stockpot, bring the coconut milk and ⅓ cup of water to a boil over high heat. Stir in the quinoa, ginger, chia seeds, and garlic, then top with the kale (you may have to add it in batches, but it will cook down). Cover, reduce heat to medium-low, and cook until the quinoa is nearly tender, about 22 minutes. Remove from the heat and let stand covered for 5 minutes to complete the cooking process.

2. Add the pineapple, lime juice, soy sauce, and salt to the quinoa-kale mixture and stir well. Adjust the seasoning, and serve warm or at room temperature.

Per serving: 280 calories, 9 g total fat, 4 g saturated fat, 0 g trans fat, 0 mg cholesterol, 580 mg sodium, 43 g total carbohydrate, 6 g dietary fiber, 7 g sugars, 10 g protein

GREEN TEA CHICKEN AND GRAPE SALAD

This twist on a classic has a creamy (but not high-calorie) consistency, thanks to a velvety mix of fat-free yogurt, chia gel, and a small amount of mayonnaise. Another plus: green tea. I'm always trying to sneak more antioxidant-rich ingredients into my diet, and the tea gives the chicken a light, fragrant flavor.

Makes four 1-cup servings

*1 pound boneless, skinless organic chicken breast, cut into
    ½-inch cubes*

*3 cups unsweetened freshly brewed green tea or jasmine green tea
    (made with 3 tea bags), chilled*

1¾ teaspoons sea salt, or to taste

*3 tablespoons plain fat-free Icelandic or Greek yogurt, such as
    Smári Organic Icelandic Yogurt—Pure*

2 tablespoons Chia Gel (page 157)

*2 tablespoons mayonnaise, such as Follow Your Heart Organic
    Vegenaise or Sir Kensington's Classic Mayonnaise (which is
    non-GMO)*

2 teaspoons fresh lemon juice

½ teaspoon freshly ground black pepper, or to taste

1 cup red or green seedless grapes, thinly sliced

1 medium stalk celery, thinly sliced

⅓ cup finely diced red onion

¼ cup sliced almonds or chopped walnuts, toasted

1 tablespoon black chia seeds

1. In a large saucepan over high heat, bring the chicken and the tea just to a boil. Add 1 teaspoon of the salt, reduce the heat to medium-low, and simmer until the chicken is cooked through, about 6 minutes. Drain the chicken well.

2. In a large bowl, stir together the yogurt, chia gel, mayonnaise, lemon juice, and pepper until well combined. Add the tea-poached

chicken cubes, grapes, celery, onion, and the remaining ¾ teaspoon of salt and stir to combine. Cover and chill in the refrigerator until ready to serve.

3. Stir in the almonds and chia seeds and serve. This salad is delicious eaten as is or enjoyed along with gluten-free caraway crackers.

Per serving: 250 calories, 11 g total fat, 1.5 g saturated fat, 0 g trans fat, 65 mg cholesterol, 620 mg sodium, 12 g total carbohydrate, 3 g dietary fiber, 7 g sugars, 26 g protein.

· ·

ORANGE-CHIA RICE SALAD WITH FRESH MINT

Generally I make vinaigrettes with chia gel, but the vinaigrette I use here works particularly well with just the seeds. The dressing is very light—you don't want to drown out all that wonderful fresh mint!—and the seeds give the citrusy rice that pleasurable little chia crunch.

Makes five 1-cup servings

1 cup short-grain brown rice
1 teaspoon sea salt, or to taste
¾ teaspoon freshly ground black pepper, or to taste
1 cup finely diced unpeeled English or Persian cucumber or peeled
   and seeded regular cucumber
2 scallions, green and white parts, thinly sliced on the diagonal
3 tablespoons chopped fresh mint
1 recipe Orange-Chia Vinaigrette (recipe follows)
1 teaspoon grated orange zest, for garnish

1. Cook the rice according to the package directions. Transfer to a medium bowl, season with the salt and pepper, and set aside to cool for about 30 minutes, stirring occasionally to help prevent sticking. Place in the refrigerator until chilled.

2. Add the cucumber, scallions, mint, and vinaigrette to the chilled rice and stir to combine. Adjust the seasonings, garnish with the orange zest, and serve.

Per serving: 180 calories, 4.5 g total fat, 1 g saturated fat, 0 g trans fat, 0 mg cholesterol, 530 mg sodium, 36 g total carbohydrate, 3 g dietary fiber, 2 g sugars, 3 g protein.

ORANGE-CHIA VINAIGRETTE

Makes about ½ cup

⅓ cup fresh orange juice
1 tablespoon extra-virgin olive oil
2 teaspoons black or white chia seeds
1 teaspoon grated orange zest
¼ teaspoon freshly ground black pepper, or to taste
⅛ teaspoon sea salt, or to taste

In a medium bowl, whisk together all of the ingredients. Let stand for about 20 minutes before serving.

CHIA CAESAR KALE SALAD

Just think, until recently, most of us only ate kale cooked . . . and then suddenly kale salad became a restaurant staple. I'm in love with kale salads and particularly like the Caesar variation—which tastes a lot like a traditional Caesar salad but is a whole lot better for you (and the heartier kale makes it extra satisfying). The kale leaves will become a little softer when they sit in the dressing for 10 minutes. You can also soften the leaves up by massaging the dressing into the kale.

Makes four 2½-cup servings

8 cups packed fresh baby kale or chopped kale leaves, thick stems removed
1 recipe Chia Caesar Dressing (recipe follows)

2 ounces small gluten-free organic crackers, such as Mary's Gone Crackers Organic—Original flavor
¼ cup grated Parmigiano-Reggiano or Pecorino Romano cheese
¼ teaspoon freshly ground black pepper, or to taste
4 lemon wedges, for garnish

1. In a large bowl, toss together the kale, dressing, and half of the crackers until well combined. Let stand about 10 minutes. Add the cheese and black pepper and toss again.

2. Arrange the salad on a platter or four plates, top with the remaining crackers, and serve with the lemon wedges on the side.

Per serving: 170 calories, 8 g total fat, 1.5 g saturated fat, 0 g trans fat, 5 mg cholesterol, 410 mg sodium, 20 g total carbohydrate, 3 g dietary fiber, 1 g sugars, 6 g protein.

CHIA CAESAR DRESSING

Makes ⅔ cup

⅓ cup Chia Gel (page 157)
2 tablespoons grainy Dijon mustard, regular or spicy
2 large garlic cloves, chopped
1 tablespoon vegetarian Worcestershire sauce
1 tablespoon fresh lemon juice
1 tablespoon extra-virgin olive oil
¼ teaspoon freshly ground black pepper, or to taste

In a blender, purée all the ingredients together until smooth. Adjust the seasoning. Use immediately or store covered in the refrigerator for up to 1 week.

DILL ROASTED CARROT AND BASMATI SALAD

Roasting carrots until they're caramelized turns an everyday vegetable into something entirely new tasting. Mixed with fragrant basmati and dill, they take rice salad to new heights!

Makes four 1-cup servings

1 cup brown basmati rice
1½ teaspoons grated lemon zest
¾ teaspoon sea salt, or to taste
2 large carrots, peeled or scrubbed, very thinly sliced crosswise
    (about ⅛ inch thick)
2½ tablespoons extra-virgin olive oil
2 tablespoons chopped fresh dill
¼ teaspoon freshly ground black pepper, or to taste
2 scallions, green and white parts, thinly sliced
1 tablespoon black chia seeds
4 lemon wedges, for garnish

1. Cook the basmati rice according to the package directions. Transfer to a medium bowl and stir in the lemon zest and ¼ teaspoon of the salt. Set aside to cool for about 30 minutes, stirring occasionally to help prevent sticking. Chill in the refrigerator.

2. Preheat the oven to 450°F.

3. Add the carrots to a large baking pan. Drizzle with 1 tablespoon of the oil, toss to coat, and arrange in a single layer. Roast until the carrots are just tender and lightly caramelized, about 12 minutes. Remove from the oven and add the dill, ¼ teaspoon of the salt, and the pepper; toss to combine.

4. Add the roasted carrots mixture and the scallions, the chia seeds, the remaining 1½ tablespoons of the oil, and the remaining ¼ teaspoon of the salt to the chilled rice and stir to combine. Adjust the seasoning and serve with the lemon wedges on the side.

Per serving: 250 calories, 11 g total fat, 1.5 g saturated fat, 0 g trans fat, 0 mg cholesterol, 460 mg sodium, 37 g total carbohydrate, 4 g dietary fiber, 3 g sugars, 4 g protein.

MESCLUN SALAD WITH PEAR, WALNUTS, AND GOAT CHEESE

This salad is lovely with walnuts or pecans, whichever you prefer (though walnuts will net you more omega-3s). To toast the nuts, either place them on a baking sheet in a 350°F oven or in a skillet over medium heat for about 10 minutes, stirring occasionally to keep them from getting too dark on one side.

Makes four 2½-cup servings

8 cups packed mesclun or mixed baby greens
1 Bosc or Anjou pear, cored, halved, and thinly sliced
⅓ cup very thinly sliced red onion
1 recipe Chia Balsamic Vinaigrette (recipe follows)
⅓ cup walnuts or pecans, toasted
1½ ounces crumbled soft goat cheese
¼ teaspoon freshly ground black pepper, or to taste

1. In a large bowl, toss together the mesclun, pear, onion, and half the vinaigrette.

2. Arrange the salad on a platter or four plates. Top with the walnuts and goat cheese, sprinkle with pepper to taste, and serve with the remaining vinaigrette on the side.

Per serving: 210 calories, 19 g total fat, 3.5 g saturated fat, 0 g trans fat, 5 mg cholesterol, 240 mg sodium, 10 g total carbohydrate, 3 g dietary fiber, 4 g sugars, 5 g protein.

CHIA BALSAMIC VINAIGRETTE

Makes ½ cup

3 tablespoons extra-virgin olive oil
3 tablespoons aged balsamic vinegar
3 tablespoons Chia Gel (page 157)
¼ cup chopped or very thinly sliced red onion
¼ teaspoon sea salt, or to taste
¼ teaspoon freshly ground black pepper, or to taste

In a blender, purée all the ingredients until smooth. Adjust the seasonings. Use immediately or store covered in the refrigerator for up to 1 week.

DINNER

. . . .

SOFT FISH TACOS WITH CHIA PICO DE GALLO

Living close to the Mexican border, I get my fair share of tacos, so I know what I'm talking about when I say these are a standout version— and so much more energizing than the greasy, cheesy fried-shell variety. You can also make this recipe with boneless, skinless chicken breasts fillets instead of fish. They're topped with pico de gallo, a salsa, made with freshly chopped ingredients.

Makes four 2-taco servings

½ cup packed fresh cilantro leaves
Juice of 1 lime (2 tablespoons)
2 large garlic cloves
¾ teaspoon sea salt, or to taste
½ teaspoon ground cumin
½ teaspoon ground coriander
1½ teaspoons extra-virgin olive oil
2 (7-ounce) farm-raised barramundi or tilapia fillets
1 Hass avocado, pitted, peeled, and sliced
8 (6-inch) soft organic corn tortillas, such as Food for Life Sprouted
* Corn Tortillas, warmed*
1 cup finely shredded red cabbage
1 recipe Chia Pico de Gallo (recipe follows)

1. In a food processor, pulse the cilantro, lime juice, garlic, ½ teaspoon of the salt, the cumin, and the coriander until well combined. Alternatively, grind these ingredients with a mortar and pestle. Set aside.

2. In a large (PFOA-free) nonstick skillet, heat the oil over medium-high heat. Cook the barramundi fillets until done, about 3 minutes per side. Slice the fillets into bite-size pieces, return to the warm skillet, and gently toss with the reserved cilantro mixture.

3. Sprinkle the avocado slices with the remaining ¼ teaspoon of

salt. Divide the barramundi slices among the tortillas and top with the cabbage and avocado. Place two tacos on each of four plates, and serve with the pico de gallo on the side.

Per serving: 290 calories, 10 g total fat, 1 g saturated fat, 0 g trans fat, 40 mg cholesterol, 650 mg sodium, 31 g total carbohydrate, 7 g dietary fiber, 3 g sugars, 25 g protein.

CHIA PICO DE GALLO

Makes 1½ cups

> 2 medium vine-ripened tomatoes, pulp and core removed
>   and finely diced
> ¼ cup finely diced white onion
> 2 tablespoons Chia Gel (page 157)
> 1 small serrano pepper, with some of the seeds, minced
> 1 tablespoon finely chopped fresh cilantro
> ¼ teaspoon sea salt, or to taste
> 2 teaspoons fresh lime juice

In a medium bowl, combine all of the ingredients. Adjust the seasonings and serve, or store covered in the refrigerator for up to 5 days.

ASIAN PAN-SEARED CHIA-CRUSTED SALMON WITH SPINACH

Salmon and chia—that's one beautiful couple! So many omega-3s in one dish. Add in the spinach, which here is served uncooked (it will wilt slightly under the heat of the salmon), and you've got an amazingly nutritious and delicious meal.

Makes four servings

4 wild center-cut salmon fillets (6 ounces each) with skin
1 recipe Asian Chia Marinade (recipe follows)
4 packed cups (4 ounces) fresh baby spinach
2 teaspoons black or white chia seeds (or 1 teaspoon of each)
¼ teaspoon sea salt, or to taste

1. Place the salmon in a baking dish and using ¼ cup of the marinade, coat the entire surface of each fillet. Let marinate for 15 minutes.

2. Spritz a large (PFOA-free) nonstick skillet with cooking spray and place over medium-high heat. In batches (2 fillets at a time), cook the salmon skin-side down for 3 minutes; reduce the heat to medium, carefully flip over each fillet, and cook until medium doneness, about 3 minutes.

3. Place the spinach on a platter and top with the salmon. Drizzle with the remaining ¼ cup of marinade, sprinkle each fillet with the chia seeds and salt, and serve.

Per serving: 300 calories, 13 g total fat, 2 g saturated fat, O g trans fat, 520 mg sodium, 10 g total carbohydrate, 2 g dietary fiber, 6 g sugars, 35 g protein.

ASIAN CHIA MARINADE

Makes ½ cup

3 tablespoons brown rice vinegar
2 tablespoons Chia Gel (page 157)
1 tablespoon tamari soy sauce
1 tablespoon honey or agave nectar
1½ teaspoons freshly grated ginger
1 teaspoon toasted sesame oil

In a small bowl, whisk together all of the ingredients. Use immediately, or cover and chill in the refrigerator for up to 2 weeks.

. . . .

INDIAN-SPICED TURKEY BURGERS
WITH CHIA CURRY KETCHUP

Turns out, those most all-American of foods—burgers—work well with Indian flavors. Here they're served without buns, but feel free to sandwich them between a crusty roll if you like, or wrap them in hearty leaves of romaine lettuce if you want to cut some carbs. Serve with Chia Sweet Potato "Fries" (page 179).

Makes four servings

1 pound lean ground organic turkey (about 94% lean)
⅓ cup grated red onion
1 tablespoon milled (ground) chia seeds
1 tablespoon finely chopped fresh cilantro
1½ teaspoons freshly grated ginger
¾ teaspoon sea salt
2 cups packed mixed Asian lettuces or mixed baby greens (2 ounces)
1 recipe Chia Curry Ketchup (recipe follows)

1. Preheat and lightly brush a grill with oil or spritz a grill pan with cooking spray.

2. In a medium bowl, gently combine the turkey, onion, milled chia seeds, cilantro, ginger, and salt. Form into 4 (4½-inch-wide) patties.

3. Grill the patties over medium-high heat until well done, about 5 minutes per side, flipping only once, if possible.

4. Arrange the lettuces on a platter or on four individual plates. Place the patties on top and drizzle with half of the ketchup. Serve with the remaining ketchup on the side.

Per serving: 210 calories, 8 g total fat, 2 g saturated fat, 0 g trans fat, 65 mg cholesterol, 660 mg sodium, 10 g total carbohydrate, 3 g dietary fiber, 4 g sugars, 23 g protein.

CHIA CURRY KETCHUP

Makes ½ cup

*¼ cup ketchup, such as Sir Kensington's Classic Ketchup or
    Annie's
Naturals Organic Ketchup
2 tablespoons Chia Gel (page 157)
2 tablespoons mango nectar, such as R.W. Knudsen Organic
    Mango Nectar
1 teaspoon apple cider vinegar
1 teaspoon freshly grated ginger
¾ teaspoon hot Madras curry powder, or to taste
½ teaspoon freshly ground black pepper, or to taste*

In a small bowl, stir all the ingredients together with a
fork. Adjust the seasonings and serve, or store covered in the
refrigerator for up to 2 weeks.

CHIA SWEET POTATO "FRIES"

I'm a big fan of sweet potatoes, a great source of vitamins A and C.
Tossing the strips with a little olive oil allows the chia seeds to stick
and gives the "fries" (which are actually baked) cute little freckles.
These also taste delicious tossed with flavored salts; just swap out the
sea salt for your favorite.

Makes four servings

*1½ pounds (about 4 medium) sweet potatoes or garnet yams, peeled
    and cut into ½-inch-wide slices, then into ½-inch strips
1½ tablespoons extra-virgin olive oil
2 tablespoons black chia seeds
½ teaspoon sea salt, or to taste*

1. Preheat the oven to 500°F.

2. In a medium bowl, toss the sweet potatoes with the olive oil. Add the chia seeds and salt and toss again to coat.

3. Spread the sweet potatoes on a nonstick baking sheet or one that has been lightly oiled. Bake until tender and golden brown, turning occasionally, about 25 to 30 minutes. Adjust salt if necessary and serve.

Per serving: 160 calories, 7 g total fat, 1 g saturated fat, O mg cholesterol, 330 mg sodium, 24 g total carbohydrate, 5 g dietary fiber, 7 g sugars, 3 g protein.

. . . .

VEGGIE TOSTADA STACK WITH EGG AND AVOCADO

This twist on a Mexican classic is super simple to make, even though it looks like you slaved in the kitchen all afternoon. Don't worry about timing everything perfectly here; you can keep the beans and sautéed veggies warm in a 200°F oven or on a warm burner.

Makes four servings

8 (6-inch) soft organic corn tortillas, such as Food for Life Sprouted Corn Tortillas, warmed

4 teaspoons extra-virgin olive oil

2 cups (6 ounces) sliced fresh cremini (baby bella) mushrooms

1 large zucchini, thinly sliced crosswise

¼ cup bottled salsa or Chia Pico de Gallo (page 176)

1 teaspoon finely chopped fresh oregano

½ teaspoon sea salt, or to taste

1 15-ounce can vegetarian refried black beans, such as Amy's Organic Refried Black Beans

2 tablespoons Chia Gel (page 157)

4 large organic eggs

½ Hass avocado, pitted, peeled, and sliced

1 teaspoon black chia seeds

1. Preheat the oven to 450°F. Spritz both sides of the tortillas with cooking spray. Place on a baking sheet and bake until crisp and lightly browned, about 5 minutes per side. Remove from the oven and set aside to cool on the pan.

2. In a medium (PFOA-free) nonstick skillet, heat 2 teaspoons of the oil over medium-high heat. Add the mushrooms and zucchini and sauté until the zucchini is softened, about 7 minutes. Add the salsa, oregano, and ¼ teaspoon of the salt and sauté for 1 minute. Cover and set aside.

3. In a small pot, warm the beans over medium heat until they start to bubble. Turn off the heat and stir the chia gel into the warm beans. Cover and set aside.

4. In a large (PFOA-free) nonstick skillet or griddle, heat the remaining 2 teaspoons of the oil over medium-high heat. Add the eggs and fry about 2 minutes on the first side and 30 seconds on the flip side for over-easy eggs. Sprinkle with the remaining ¼ teaspoon of salt.

5. Spread the bean mixture over each crisp tortilla, about ¼ cup per tortilla. Top with the vegetable mixture, about ¼ cup per tortilla. Stack 2 tortillas on top of each other, creating 4 stacks of 2 tortillas each. Top each stack with a fried egg, avocado slices, and a sprinkling of chia seeds. Adjust the seasonings and serve warm.

Per serving: 370 calories, 15 g total fat, 3 g saturated fat, 185 mg cholesterol, 660 mg sodium, 45 g total carbohydrate, 12 g dietary fiber, 4 g sugars, 17 g protein.

• •

CHICKEN CHIA CHILI

Hopefully you'll have some of this left over for lunch: it tastes even better the next day (it freezes well, too—just add the avocado at serving time). If you prefer, you can also make this dish with lean ground turkey. Serve with warm soft corn tortillas or corn tortilla chips.

Makes six 1⅓-cup servings

1 tablespoon extra-virgin olive oil

1 pound ground organic chicken breast

1 large red onion (about 1½ cups), diced

1 small jalapeño pepper, with or without seeds, minced

3 large garlic cloves, minced

1 32-ounce carton low-sodium organic chicken broth

1 14.5-ounce can (1¾ cups) crushed fire-roasted organic tomatoes

¼ cup black or white chia seeds

Juice and zest of 1 lime (2 tablespoons juice)

1½ tablespoons chili powder

1 teaspoon sea salt, or to taste

1 15-ounce can low-sodium organic Great Northern or cannellini
   beans, drained, or 1½ cups cooked dried beans

3 tablespoons chopped fresh cilantro

½ Hass avocado, pitted, peeled, and diced

1. In a large stockpot, heat the oil over medium-high heat. Add the chicken, onion, and jalapeño, and sauté until the chicken is cooked through and crumbly, about 6 minutes. Stir in the garlic and sauté for 1 minute more.

2. Add the broth, tomatoes, chia seeds, lime juice, chili powder, and salt and bring to a boil over high heat. Reduce heat to low, cover, and simmer, stirring occasionally, for 45 minutes.

3. Stir in the beans and half of the cilantro and simmer, uncovered, over low heat, stirring occasionally, until desired consistency, about 30 minutes more. Adjust the seasonings.

4. Spoon the chili into bowls and top with the avocado, the remaining cilantro, and the lime zest. Serve hot.

Per serving: 260 calories, 9 g total fat, 1.5 g saturated fat, 0 g trans fat, 40 mg cholesterol, 700 mg sodium, 24 g total carbohydrate, 8 g dietary fiber, 5 g sugars, 23 g protein.

BROCCOLI VELVET SOUP

When I was growing up, you pretty much had only one liquid you could add to give food a creamy texture—cream (or milk). Now, with so many plant-based milks on the market, it's easy to find a healthful replacement. And neither flavor nor texture suffers for it. You'll see when you try this soup—it really does taste like there's cream in it!

Makes four 1½-cup servings

1 tablespoon extra-virgin olive oil

1 large white onion, chopped

1 small serrano pepper, with some of the seeds, minced

1 teaspoon apple cider vinegar

¾ teaspoon sea salt, or to taste

3 tablespoons garbanzo bean (chickpea) flour or gluten-free
all-purpose baking flour, such as Bob's Red Mill Gluten-Free
All-Purpose Baking Flour

2½ cups plain unsweetened almond milk or other plant-based milk

2 cups low-sodium vegetable broth

8 ounces roughly chopped fresh broccoli florets with tender stems

2 tablespoons white chia seeds

⅛ teaspoon freshly grated or ground nutmeg, or to taste, plus more
for garnish

1. In a large stockpot, heat the oil over medium-high heat. Add the onion, serrano pepper, vinegar, and ¼ teaspoon of the salt and sauté until the onion is softened, about 5 minutes.

2. In a liquid measuring cup or a small bowl, whisk together the flour and ¼ cup of the almond milk until smooth.

3. Stir the flour-milk mixture, the remaining 2¼ cups of almond milk, and the broth into the onion mixture. Add the broccoli, chia seeds, nutmeg, and the remaining ½ teaspoon of salt and bring just to a boil over medium-high heat. Reduce the heat to low and simmer,

covered, until the broccoli is very tender, about 25 minutes, stirring a couple of times while simmering.

4. In a blender, carefully purée the soup in batches using the hot-fill line as a guide. Adjust the seasonings and reheat, if necessary. Ladle the soup into individual bowls, sprinkle with additional nutmeg if desired, and serve.

Per serving: 160 calories, 7 g total fat, 1 g saturated fat, 0 g trans fat, 0 mg cholesterol, 620 mg sodium, 20 g total carbohydrate, 6 g dietary fiber, 8 g sugars, 4 g protein.

• •

CORIANDER LENTILS AND KALE

Greens and legumes are a time-honored team, and the combination of the two—with all the fiber and protein they bring to the table—makes this dish amazingly satisfying. Serve over rice, if you like.

Makes four 1-rounded-cup servings

1 tablespoon extra-virgin olive oil
1 medium yellow or white onion (about 1 cup), diced
1 medium carrot, scrubbed and finely diced
Juice and zest of ½ lemon (1½ tablespoons juice)
¾ teaspoon sea salt, or to taste
2 large garlic cloves, minced
1 32-ounce carton low-sodium vegetable broth
¾ cup dry lentils, rinsed and drained
2 tablespoons black or white chia seeds
¾ teaspoon ground coriander or cumin, or to taste
½ teaspoon freshly ground black pepper, or to taste
4 cups (4 ounces) packed fresh baby kale or chopped kale, thick stems
*   removed*
½ cup plain fat-free Icelandic or Greek yogurt, such as Smári
*   Organic Icelandic Yogurt—Pure*
2 tablespoons roughly chopped fresh cilantro

1. In a large stockpot heat the oil over medium-high heat. Add the onion, carrot, lemon juice, and ¼ teaspoon of the salt and sauté until the onion is softened, about 5 minutes. Add the garlic and sauté until fragrant, about 30 seconds.

2. Add the broth, lentils, chia seeds, coriander, pepper, and the remaining ½ teaspoon of salt and bring to a boil over high heat. Reduce heat to medium-low, stir in the kale and simmer, partially covered, until the lentils are tender, about 28 minutes. Adjust the seasoning.

3. Ladle the mixture into individual bowls; top with the yogurt, lemon zest, and cilantro; and serve.

Per serving: 240 calories, 6 g total fat, 1 g saturated fat, 600 mg sodium, 35 g total carbohydrate, 13 g dietary fiber, 7 g sugars, 15 g protein.

. . . .

BEET AND GOAT CHEESE SALAD

This past year I couldn't get enough beets—I'd make a beeline for them as soon as I hit the farmers' market. They just looked so gorgeous stacked up on the vendors' tables. This salad works with the beets served warm or, if you prefer to roast them in advance and store in the refrigerator, chilled.

Makes four approximately 1-cup servings

> 4 medium beets, roasted, peeled, and thinly sliced
>   (see page 186)
> ⅛ teaspoon sea salt, or to taste
> ¼ cup Chia Balsamic Vinaigrette (page 174) or balsamic vinaigrette
>   of choice
> 3 ounces soft goat cheese, crumbled
> 1 teaspoon black chia seeds
> 1 tablespoon tiny fresh basil leaves or chopped fresh basil
> ¼ teaspoon freshly ground black pepper, or to taste

Arrange the beets on a platter or divide among four plates. Sprinkle with the salt, vinaigrette, goat cheese, chia seeds, basil, and black pepper, and serve.

Per serving: 130 calories, 8 g total fat, 3.5 g saturated fat, 0 g trans fat, 10 mg cholesterol, 260 mg sodium, 9 g total carbohydrate, 2 g dietary fiber, 7 g sugars, 5 g protein.

ROASTING BEETS

Individually wrap unpeeled medium beets in aluminum foil (recycled, if you can find it). Roast in a 375°F oven until the beets can be easily pierced with a knife, about 1 hour. Unwrap. When the beets are cool enough to handle, peel off the skins—they should slip right off. Note: You may want to wear rubber gloves since the beets (presuming you're using red ones, though golden work nicely in this recipe, too) will stain your hands.

THAI BASIL VEGGIE FRIED RICE

Remember to make the rice in advance and chill it. If you start with warm rice, the fried rice may become a bit too mushy. I like pineapple in fried rice, but if you have other fruit on hand, give it a try . . . just make sure its texture will hold up: apples, pears, and grapes do well.

Makes four 1-cup servings

2 tablespoons unrefined coconut oil, such as Nutiva Organic Extra Virgin Coconut Oil
1 small or ½ large white onion (about ½ cup), finely chopped
2 cups bite-size pieces cauliflower florets
3 large garlic cloves, minced
1 small serrano pepper, with some of the seeds, minced

½ cup finely diced fresh pineapple, drained

3 cups cooked brown basmati rice, chilled

1 tablespoon natural ketchup, such as Annie's Naturals Organic
  Ketchup

¾ teaspoon sea salt, or to taste

2 scallions, green and white parts, thinly sliced

¼ cup chopped fresh Thai basil or other basil

1 tablespoon black chia seeds

2 teaspoons tamari soy sauce, or to taste

1. In a wok or extra-large (PFOA-free) nonstick skillet, heat the oil over medium-high heat.

2. Add the onion and stir-fry until lightly browned, about 4 minutes.

3. Add the cauliflower, garlic, and serrano pepper and stir-fry for 2 minutes.

4. Add the pineapple, chilled rice, ketchup, and salt and stir-fry until the rice begins to caramelize and the cauliflower is just cooked through, about 7 minutes.

5. Add the scallions, basil, chia seeds, and soy sauce and stir-fry for 1 minute. Serve immediately.

Per serving: 280 calories, 9 g total fat, 6 g saturated fat, 0 g trans fat, 650 mg sodium, 44 g total carbohydrate, 6 g dietary fiber, 5 g sugars, 6 g protein.

SNACKS AND DESSERTS

. . . .

CHIA EDAMAME DIP

This dip is best pureed in a food processor or a very powerful blender. If you only have a regular blender, you may need to add a little more of the cooking liquid, which will net you a thinner dip (it will still taste yummy, though!). Serve with gluten-free crackers.

Makes eight ½-cup servings

> *1 10-ounce bag frozen shelled organic edamame*
> *Juice of 1 lemon (3 tablespoons)*
> *2 tablespoons Chia Gel (page 157)*
> *2 tablespoons tahini (sesame seed paste)*
> *1 large garlic clove, chopped, or to taste*
> *¾ teaspoon sea salt, or to taste*
> *⅛ teaspoon cayenne pepper, or to taste*

1. Boil the edamame according to the package directions. Drain, and reserve 1 cup of the cooking liquid.

2. In a food processor, blend the edamame, lemon juice, chia gel, tahini, garlic, salt, cayenne, and ⅓ cup of the reserved cooking liquid until smooth, at least 2 minutes, adding extra cooking liquid, only as needed, for desired consistency. Adjust the seasoning.

3. Spoon into a serving bowl and serve immediately, or cover and store in the refrigerator until ready to use.

Per serving: 70 calories, 4 g total fat, 0.5 g saturated fat, 0 g trans fat, 0 mg cholesterol, 220 mg sodium, 5 g total carbohydrate, 2 g dietary fiber, 1 g sugars, 5 g protein.

CHIA GUACAMOLE

This Mexican classic can be made many different ways, so don't feel you have to adhere to this recipe to the letter. Some people like to add cumin and cayenne; others prefer to use hot sauce or jalapeño peppers instead of serranos. Some like white onion; I'm partial to red. If it suits your fancy, add a little pressed garlic. I like to throw in tomato for color and an added shot of vitamin C, but if it's off-season and the tomatoes look more like rubber balls than luscious produce, there's no harm in skipping it altogether.

Makes six ⅓-cup servings

2 medium ripe Hass avocados, peeled, seeded, and cut in half
1 medium vine-ripened tomato, seeds removed and diced
½ cup finely diced red onion
½ serrano chile pepper with seeds, or more to taste, finely chopped
¼ cup chopped fresh cilantro
3 tablespoons Chia Gel (page 157)
2 teaspoons fresh lime juice, or to taste
½ teaspoon sea salt, or to taste

1. In a medium bowl, mash the avocados with a fork just until lumpy, not smooth.

2. Add the tomato, onion, serrano pepper, cilantro, chia gel, lime juice, and salt and stir until well combined. Taste and adjust the seasonings. Serve with baked tortilla chips or Soft Fish Tacos with Chia Pico de Gallo (page 175).

Per serving: 90 calories, 7 g total fat, 1 g saturated fat, 0 g trans fat, 0 mg cholesterol, 200 mg sodium, 6 g total carbohydrate, 4 g dietary fiber, 1 g sugars, 1 g protein.

CHIA WHITE CHOCOLATE MACADAMIA COOKIES

Here you have the best of both cookie worlds—crisp *and* chewy. Car-melization is key, so bake the cookies 1 minute longer than you think you need to.

Makes sixteen 1-cookie servings

> 1 tablespoon white or black chia seeds
> 1 cup gluten-free all-purpose baking flour, such as Bob's Red Mill Gluten-Free All-Purpose Baking Flour
> 1 teaspoon baking soda
> ½ teaspoon sea salt
> ¼ teaspoon ground cinnamon
> ⅓ cup unrefined virgin coconut oil, such as Nutiva Organic Extra Virgin Coconut Oil
> 1 cup organic raw sugar
> 2 tablespoons unsweetened applesauce
> 1½ teaspoons pure vanilla extract
> ½ cup gluten-free old-fashioned oats, such as Bob's Red Mill Gluten-Free Old Fashioned Rolled Oats
> 4 ounces high-quality white chocolate chunks or chips
> ½ cup chopped unsalted macadamia nuts

1. In a small bowl, whisk the chia seeds together with 3 table-spoons of room-temperature purified water. Set aside.

2. Preheat the oven to 375°F. Line two baking sheets with unbleached parchment paper. Set aside.

3. In a medium bowl, combine the flour, baking soda, salt, and cinnamon. Set aside.

4. In a large bowl, stir together the oil and sugar until combined. Stir in the chia mixture, applesauce, and vanilla until well combined.

5. Stir the flour mixture into the oil-sugar mixture until blended. Stir in the oats, then the white chocolate chunks and nuts until evenly mixed.

6. Drop the dough onto the baking sheets, 8 cookies each, using about 2 rounded tablespoons of dough per cookie. Bake until browned, about 15 to 17 minutes.

7. Remove from the oven and let the cookies stand for 10 minutes on the cookie sheets to firm. Transfer the cookies to cooling racks to crisp for at least 10 minutes and serve. (You can also store the cookies in a covered airtight container in the freezer for later use.)

Per serving: 200 calories, 10 g total fat, 6 g saturated fat, 0 g trans fat, 0 mg cholesterol, 160 mg sodium, 27 g total carbohydrate, 2 g dietary fiber, 19 g sugars, 2 g protein.

. . . .

CHIA CHERRY VANILLA SMOOTHIE

If it's cherry season, you're in luck; just use a cherry pitter to remove the pits. Otherwise, frozen pitted cherries work very nicely, too.

Makes two 1-cup servings

1¼ cups fresh Bing (sweet) cherries, pitted and chilled
1 cup vanilla organic frozen yogurt or dairy-free dessert
⅓ cup plain unsweetened almond milk or other plant-based milk, chilled
3 tablespoons Chia Gel (page 157)
2 teaspoons fresh lemon juice
¼ teaspoon pure vanilla extract

In a blender, blend all the ingredients together until smooth. Pour into two tall chilled glasses and serve.

Per serving: 180 calories, 4 g total fat, 1.5 g saturated fat, 0 g trans fat, 10 mg cholesterol, 60 mg sodium, 35 g total carbohydrate, 3 g dietary fiber, 27 g sugars, 4 g protein.

. . . .

CHIA OAT APPLE CRISP

In summer, this recipe translates nicely to berry and stone fruit crisps. Just toss the fruit with a little flour or cornstarch before adding the topping to soak up the juices and prevent the dessert from becoming too runny.

Makes six approximately ½-cup servings

> ⅓ cup gluten-free all-purpose baking flour, such as Bob's Red Mill
>   Gluten-Free All-Purpose Baking Flour
> 2 tablespoons organic brown sugar
> Pinch of sea salt (skip if you're using salted vegan butter)
> 2 tablespoons organic raw sugar
> 4 tablespoons (½ stick) vegan butter, such as Earth Balance, or
>   unsalted butter, cold and cut into small cubes
> ½ cup gluten-free old-fashioned oats, such as Bob's Red Mill
>   Gluten-Free Old Fashioned Rolled Oats
> 1 tablespoon black or white chia seeds
> 1½ pounds apples (about 4 apples), such as Gala or Fuji, peeled,
>   cored, and cut into ¼-inch or ½-inch slices
> Juice of ½ small lemon (1 tablespoon)
> ½ teaspoon ground cinnamon

1. Preheat the oven to 375°F. Lightly coat an 8-inch-square baking dish with cooking spray. Set aside.

2. In a medium bowl, stir together the flour, brown sugar, the salt (if using), and 1 tablespoon of the raw sugar. Using a pastry blender or your fingers, work the butter into the flour mixture until you have a coarse meal. Add the oats and chia seeds and work into the mixture. Set aside.

3. In a separate medium bowl, toss the apples with the lemon juice, cinnamon, and the remaining 1 tablespoon of the raw sugar. Transfer the apple mixture to the baking dish and top with the flour-oat mixture. (If the crisp comes close to the top of the pan, place the

pan on a rimmed baking sheet to save yourself the oven cleanup.) Bake until golden brown and bubbly, about 1 hour. Serve warm.

Per serving: 215 calories, 9 g total fat, 3 g saturated fat, O g trans fat, O mg cholesterol, 85 mg sodium, 35 g total carbohydrate, 5 g dietary fiber, 21 g sugars, 2 g protein.

. . . .

CHIA CHOCOLATE PUDDING

I know what you're thinking: This woman, living on an avocado farm as she does, has gone overboard with the avos. Who has avocado for dessert? But trust me on this. Avocado lends a lovely creaminess to this pudding (not to mention throwing healthy fats, fiber, and vitamin E into the mix), and you won't even know it's there. Plus, when dessert is this healthy, forget the guilt. It's good for you!

Makes three ½-cup servings

> *1 fully ripened Hass avocado, pitted and peeled*
> *¼ cup honey or agave nectar*
> *3 tablespoons Chia Gel (page 157)*
> *2½ tablespoons unsweetened fair-trade cocoa powder*
> *½ teaspoon pure vanilla extract*
> *¼ teaspoon + ⅛ teaspoon sea salt*
> *Pinch of cayenne pepper*

1. In a food processor or the bowl of an electric mixer, blend the avocado, honey, chia gel, cocoa powder, vanilla, salt, and cayenne until creamy and fluffy, at least 2 minutes, scraping down the sides a couple of times to ensure that all the ingredients are well incorporated.

2. Transfer the mixture to two small dessert dishes and chill for at least 1 hour. This pudding is delicious served with strawberries.

Per serving: 180 calories, 8 g total fat, 1.5 g saturated fat, O g trans fat, O mg cholesterol, 300 mg sodium, 30 g total carbohydrate, 5 g dietary fiber, 23 g sugars, 2 g protein.

With Gratitude and Joy

. . . . . .

There may be only one name on the cover, but most every book is in some way a co-creative effort. And that was certainly very true in this case.

With my deepest gratitude and joy:

To my amazing collaborator, Daryn Eller. I can't imagine making this journey without you and your beautiful and talented soul by my side. No doubt, you are proof of good karma.

To my agent extraordinaire, Bonnie Solow. Thank you for always going above and beyond the call of duty and patiently teaching me the ropes. More good karma!

To Jackie Newgent, RD, your delicious and delightful knowledge made us all better. So thankful to have you part of the magic.

To Diane Bell, for your yoga expertise and inspiration, and Jeffrey Ford, for sharing your chia-powered running story. To Sarah Vollmer, for adding your delightful energy and edits to the mix.

To Leah Miller, my wonderful (and kickass) editor at Crown Publishing. I will always be grateful to you for reaching out and making all this possible *and* so much fun. Deep gratitude for your insightful feedback and awesome edits!

Many thanks to my incredible publisher, Tina Constable, who was a true believer in the magic of chia from the beginning. Not only did you come up with the idea for a book on chia, but you also had the confidence and patience to have me be the one to author it. I am so blessed to have your unwavering support.

Thank you also to editor-in-chief Mauro DiPreta, and the entire Crown team, for your consistent talent and infectious enthusiasm, especially Meredith McGowan, Tammy Blake, Lauren Cook, and Mary Anne Stewart.

Much gratitude to Heather Bandura, Karsha Chang, Barbara Marks, and Leigh Needham for your public relations prowess. It is such a joy to seed so many souls with you dynamic gals.

A big thank-you to my friends who have supported and inspired me on my journey: Greg Beattie; Eddie Bernstein; Bob Burke; Jeanne Christiansen; John Craven; Elizabeth Crook; Kara Fine; Ariana Garrett; Peter and Linda Gevorkian; Nick Giannuzzi; Wendy Gilleland; Frank and Theresa Golbeck; Seth Goldman; Stacy, David, Lev, and Shayna Grossman; Adam Haber; Mike Hannigan; Dianne Harmon; Robert Helgeson Jr.; Arno Hesse; Charles Hung; John and Ami Ken; Jeff Klein; Jeffrey Klineman; Jackie Townsend Konstanturos; Dal LaMagna; Georgia Lambert; Ray Latif; Mike Lee; Scott Leonard; Ryan Lewendon; Jim Lieb; Laura and Jay Lieberman; Chris Lindstrom; Josh Mailman; Chris Mann; Jeff Mendelsohn; Peggy and Derrell Mincey; Joyce Muraoka; Ruth Murray; Barry Nathanson; Steven and Ellen Osinski; Matt Patsky; Jamie Phillips; Gerry Ransom; Matt Reynolds; Tom Rider; Kendall Riding; Karen and John Roberts; Dale Rodriguez; Nancy Rosenzweig; Shawn Rubin; Wayne Silby; Diane Snyder; Joel Solomon; Greg Steltenpohl; Woody Tasch; Rob Thomas; Heather Van Dusen; Marco Vangelisti; Grace Venus; Mary Waldner; Bill Weiland; and Ruth and Stanley Westreich.

Heaps of gratitude to all the dedicated and talented souls on the Mamma Chia team, past and present. This really is a team sport and I am blessed to share this adventure with you. Thank you!

Love and gratitude to the Mamma Chia community. Thank you so much for taking this ride with us and helping us spread the love of chia.

To my family: Kathleen and Donald Flynn; Katie and Jeff Harvey; Jim and Barb Hawkins; Audrey and Dave Hoffman; Bruce, Donna, Marisa, Nick, and Sean Hoffman; Maureen O'Connell; Pat and Clyda O'Connell and the rest of the wonderful O'Connell clan. Your love is deeply appreciated.

To Lance, your love and kindness inspires me daily. I am so grateful for your unwavering support and friendship. I love you so!

Appendix

• • • • • •

THE *CHIA VITALITY* YOGA PRACTICE

You might remember from the initial definition of *vitality* in this book (see page 3) that vitality is not one single thing, but rather the integration of many—as is yoga. Yoga originated in India about five thousand years ago and comes from a Sanskrit word meaning "to unite." It refers to the union of body, mind, and spirit and the connection between individual consciousness and universal consciousness. Although we've come to know it mostly as a form of exercise, yoga also includes meditation and an overall philosophical outlook that emphasizes love, compassion, and oneness with the world. The ultimate purpose of yoga (in all its forms) is to expand your consciousness and gain a deeper awareness and understanding of your true nature—your soul, that is, and its true purpose. For all these reasons, yoga seems particularly compatible with the pursuit of greater vitality. I think you'll find that it can improve every aspect of your life, not to mention strengthen your alignment with your own beautiful soul!

The yoga practice in this chapter should take you about 25 minutes, but it's very flexible. In the suggested schedule on pages 153–55, I recommend that you work up to doing the whole practice. To make it shorter, do fewer repetitions of each pose, or leave out some of the poses. You can, of course, do the whole 25-minute practice right from the start if you like. Either way, as you progress, listen to your body and let the practice answer its needs.

THE VICTORIOUS VITALITY BREATH

Many forms of physical yoga allow breathing to set the rhythm of the practice. Typically, it's ujjayi breathing, and here's how you do it: Gently inhale through your nose, then with your mouth open slightly, make a *ha* sound as you exhale through your nose. Try it again, but this time with your mouth closed, so as you exhale, you hear a hissing sound and feel a slight vibration in the back of your throat.

Ujjayi means "victorious"—so apt because by calming the nervous system and increasing oxygen in the blood, that's exactly how it makes you feel! Every inhale and exhale is powerful. Use ujjayi breathing to help you as you go through the *Chia Vitality* yoga practice and at other times of the day as well. When you want to ground yourself, deflect stress, and connect more fully with the present moment, breathe. Just b-r-e-a-t-h-e.

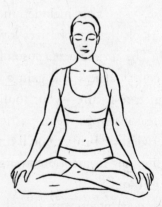

CROSS-LEGGED POSITION
Sukhasana

Take a minute to sit quietly in a cross-legged position with your hands resting, palms down, on your knees, or gently resting in your lap. Calm your thoughts and notice your breathing. Try ujjayi breathing (see above).

As you get the hang of it, use ujjayi breathing throughout the rest of the practice. Close your eyes. Begin to observe the inflow and outflow of your breath. With each inhalation and exhalation, allow yourself to become more relaxed, more comfortable, and more at ease. Now set your intention for the practice. Perhaps it is to be more kind and compassionate to yourself. Or perhaps it is to honor and listen to your body, or maybe it is to be in total gratitude. Open your eyes and begin.

Move into . . .

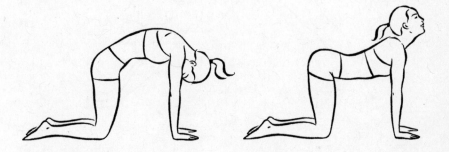

CAT-COW POSE
Marjaryasana-Bitilasana

1. Work your way onto your hands and knees, making sure that your knees are directly beneath your hips and your arms are underneath your shoulders in a straight line. Your spine, neck, and head should be in a neutral position, eyes on the floor, fingers spread.

2. As you exhale, draw your abdominal muscles in, tuck your tailbone, and round your back. Relax your neck and let your head curl inward.

3. Inhale as you come out of *cat* and move into *cow*. Roll your chest forward, lifting it toward the ceiling, and roll your sitting bones up, allowing your back to gently bend and your head to lift. Look forward.

Do 5 times.

Things to be mindful of: Throughout the asana, press your hands into the floor and roll your inner elbows forward.

Move into . . .

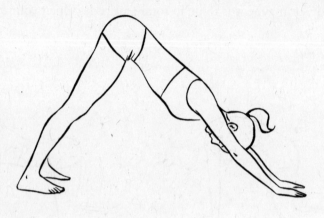

DOWNWARD-FACING DOG
Adho Mukha Svanasana

1. From a neutral hands-and-knees position, exhale, turn your toes under, and lift your knees, allowing your sitting bones to move upward and your back to lengthen. With your head between your arms, inhale and press your index fingers into the floor while rolling your inner elbows forward.

2. Draw the inside of your upper thighs up and gently stretch your calves toward the floor. Bend your knees if you feel a strain. Look toward your navel. Stay in the pose for 5 breaths, occasionally bending one knee, then the other, to loosen up your hamstrings.

Things to be mindful of: Aim to have a straight line from your hands to your hips. Don't let your chest sag toward the floor or your shoulders inch up near your ears.

Move into . . .

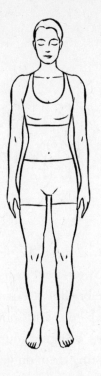

MOUNTAIN POSE

Tadasana

1. From *downward-facing dog* (*adho mukha svanasana*), inhale and walk or hop your feet between your hands. Straighten your legs, or keep them bent if that's more comfortable. Exhale and roll up through your spine until you're standing upright, legs straight with your arms at your sides. Separate your feet hip-width apart, toes pointing forward, and balance your weight between your toes and heels.

2. Roll your shoulders down your back and your chest upward. Gaze forward. Stay in the pose for 5 breaths.

Things to be mindful of: Try to elongate your upper body upward (as if a string attached to the top of your head were pulling you up) as you ground your feet and lengthen your lower body toward the floor.

Move into . . .

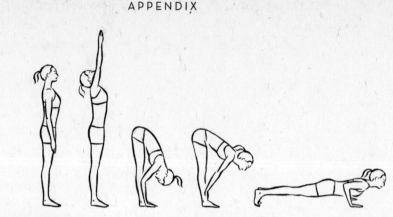

SUN SALUTATION A

Surya Namaskar A

1. From *mountain pose* (*tadasana*), bring your hands to your chest in prayer position. Inhale. Sweep your arms down then up until your palms meet overhead. Gaze briefly at your thumbs. Exhale, and with palms facing outward, sweep your arms down as you bend at the hip joints and fold over your legs, bringing your palms or fingertips to the floor next to your feet or resting them on your shins. Bend your knees if you need to.

2. Inhale and lengthen your spine forward to create a flat back, keeping your hands or fingertips on the floor or, if that strains your hamstrings, placing them on your shins. Bring your head up so your neck is in line with your spine. Gaze forward.

3. Exhale, bend your knees, walk or hop your feet back behind you, and lower to *four-limb staff pose* (*chaturanga dandasana*): Up on your toes, body parallel to the floor, bend your elbows to 90 degrees, and slowly lower your torso and legs a few inches off the ground. (Try not to allow your torso to drop below your elbows.) Draw your abdominal muscles in and hug your elbows inward to help you stay steady. If this is beyond your reach right now (and don't worry, you'll get there!), let your knees touch the floor, and then slowly lower your chest to the ground in a controlled movement.

4. Inhale and roll forward to the tops of your feet as you bring your chest upward into *upward-facing dog* (*urdhva mukha svanasana*). Supporting your weight with your hands flat, roll your shoulders down

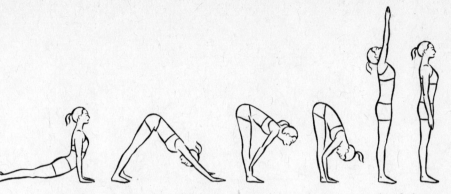

your back and broaden through your chest. Gaze upward. If this is difficult, move into *cobra* (*bhujangasana*) instead: From *four-limb staff pose* (*chaturanga dandasana*) (step 3) allow your body to come down to the floor with the tops of your feet, your thighs, and your pubic bone pressing down. As you inhale, push down on your hands and raise your upper body up, working to straighten your arms (they may straighten a little or all the way—either is fine). Roll your shoulders down your back and open through your collarbones. Gaze slightly upward.

5. Exhale, tuck your toes, and push back with your hands to raise your sitting bones and come into *downward-facing dog* (*adho mukha svanasana*). Look toward your navel. Stay in the pose for 5 breaths.

6. Inhale, bend your knees, and walk or hop your feet between your hands. Keeping your hands or fingertips on the floor or placing them on your shins, lengthen your spine forward to create a flat back. Gaze forward.

7. Exhale, fold over your legs again, then inhale, raise your arms to the side, and, with a flat back, raise your torso and bring your hands to meet above your head. Sweep your arms back down and stand in *mountain pose* (*tadasana*).

Do 4 times.

Things to be mindful of: Do this series of moves fluidly, flowing from one pose to the next. Let your inhales and exhales guide your speed. In downward-facing dog, think about lifting up through your sitting bones and down through your heels.

Move into . . .

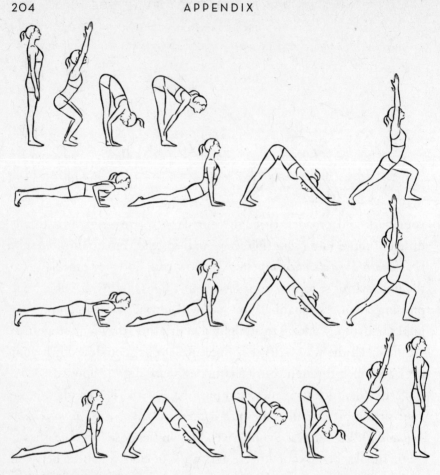

SUN SALUTATION B

Surya Namaskar B

　1. From *mountain pose* (*tadasana*), inhale, bend your knees, bring your hips down (as if you were sitting in a chair), and raise your arms above your head, elbows next to your ears. Exhale, and with palms facing outward, sweep your arms down as you bend at the hip joints and fold over your legs, bringing your palms or fingertips to the floor next to your feet or resting them on your shins. Bend your knees if you need to.

　2. Inhale and lengthen your spine forward to create a flat back, keeping your hands or fingertips on the floor or, if that strains your hamstrings, placing them on your shins. Bring your head up so your neck is in line with your spine. Gaze forward.

3. Exhale, bend your knees, walk or hop your feet back behind you, and lower to *four-limb staff pose* (*chaturanga dandasana*): Up on your toes, body parallel to the floor, bend your elbows to 90 degrees and slowly lower your torso and legs a few inches off the ground. (Try not to allow your torso to drop below your elbows.) Draw your abdominal muscles in and hug your elbows inward to help you stay steady. If this is beyond your reach right now (and don't worry, you'll get there!), let your knees touch the floor and then slowly lower your chest to the ground in a controlled movement.

4. Inhale and roll forward to the tops of your feet as you bring your chest upward into *upward-facing dog* (*urdhva mukha svanasana*). Supporting your weight with your hands flat, roll your shoulders down your back and broaden through your chest. Gaze upward. If this is difficult, move into *cobra* (*bhujangasana*) instead: From *four-limb staff pose* (*chaturanga dandasana*) allow your body to come down to the floor with the tops of your feet, your thighs, and your pubic bone pressing down. As you inhale, push down on your hands and raise your upper body up, working to straighten your arms (they may straighten a little or all the way—either is fine). Roll your shoulders down your back and open through your collarbones. Gaze slightly upward.

5. Exhale, tuck your toes, and push back with your hands to raise your sitting bones and come into *downward-facing dog* (*adho mukha svanasana*). Still exhaling, move into *warrior I* (*virabhadrasana I*): Look forward, turn your left heel in 45 to 60 degrees, and bring your right foot to the floor next to your right thumb, bending your knee at a 90-degree angle as you go. Inhale and raise your torso as you sweep your arms above your head. Gently rotate your pelvis so your hips are facing forward.

6. Exhale, place your hands on the floor on either side of your right foot, and move through *four-limb staff pose* to *upward-facing dog* (or variations), then back to *downward-facing dog*. Repeat *warrior I* (*virabhadrasana I*) on the left side.

7. When you come back to *downward-facing dog* (*adho mukha svanasana*) for the third time, stay in the pose for 5 breaths.

8. Inhale, bend your knees, and walk or hop your feet between

your hands. Keeping your hands of fingertips on the floor or placing them on your shins, lengthen your spine forward to create a flat back. Gaze forward.

9. Exhale, bend your knees, lower your hips, and raise your arms to come back into *chair pose* (*utkatasana*). Inhale, straighten your legs as you sweep your arms down, and bring your hands into prayer position at your chest. Exhale in *tadasana* (*mountain pose*).

Do 4 times.

Things to be mindful of: As with *sun salutation A* (*surya namaskar*) (page 202), do this series of moves fluidly, flowing from one pose to the next. Let your inhales and exhales guide your speed. In *warrior I* (*virabhadrasana I*), think about lowering your lunging thigh so it's parallel to the floor, being careful to keep your knee in line with your ankle.

Move into . . .

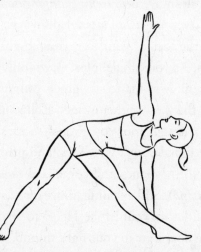

TRIANGLE POSE
Utthita Trikonasana

1. From *mountain pose* (*tadasana*) (page 201), exhale, turn to the side, and step or hop your feet 3 to 4 feet apart. Raise your arms out to the side at shoulder height, palms down. Tighten your arms and lengthen through your fingertips.

2. Inhale, turn your right foot out 90 degrees, and pivot your left foot slightly to the right. Align your right heel with the left heel. Turn your head to look at the fingers of your right hand.

3. Exhale, tuck your right hip, and bring your torso out over your right leg. Bend from your hip to bring your right hand down to rest on

your shin, ankle, or the floor. Stretch your left arm up to the ceiling so that your arms make a straight line. Gaze upward at your left hand. Stay in the pose for 5 breaths.

4. Lift out of the pose, reverse your feet, and repeat on the other side. Come back into *mountain pose* (*tadasana*).

Things to be mindful of: As you hold the pose, anchor your body by pressing your back heel to the floor. Think of lengthening both sides of your torso rather than curling over the side to reach your shin, ankle, or the floor.

Move into . . .

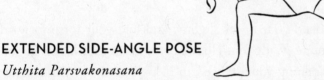

EXTENDED SIDE-ANGLE POSE
Utthita Parsvakonasana

1. Exhale, turn to the side, and step or hop your feet 3 to 4 feet apart. Raise your arms out to the side at shoulder height, palms down. Tighten your arms and lengthen through your fingertips.

2. Inhale, turn your right foot out 90 degrees, and pivot your left foot slightly to the right. Align your right heel with the left heel. Turn your head to look at the fingers of your right hand.

3. Exhale, anchor your left heel to the floor, then bend your right knee at a 90-degree angle so it's directly above your ankle and your thigh is as perpendicular to the floor as possible. Bring your right palm or fingertips to the floor beside your right foot. (If this is too challenging, rest your right elbow on your right knee.) Bring your left arm alongside your left ear, palm facing down, and reach it away from your body. Roll your chest open and turn your head toward your armpit. Stay in the pose 5 breaths.

4. Lift out of the pose, reverse your feet, and repeat on the other side.

Things to be mindful of: Push your bent knee back into your arm and pull the buttock of your bent leg in to keep your body in one plane.

Move into . . .

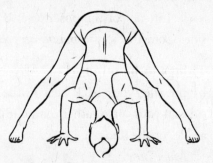

WIDE-LEGGED FORWARD BEND A
Prasarita Padottanasana A

1. Come back to *mountain pose* (*tadasana*) (page 201). Exhale, turn to the side, and step or hop your feet 3 to 4 feet apart, perhaps even wider if you're tall. Rest your hands on your hips. Inhale and lengthen up through your spine.

2. Exhale, bend your knees slightly, and fold your torso forward from the hip joints. With your elbows bent, place your hands flat on the ground (widening your stance can help you achieve this), either with your fingertips in line with your toes or, if this is too challenging, in front of your toes.

3. Inhale, press firmly through your hands, straighten your arms, and lengthen your spine forward to create a flat back. Bring your head up so your neck is in line with your spine. Exhale, bend your elbows, and fold your torso back down. If you can, place the crown of your head on the floor. Stay in this pose for 5 breaths.

4. To come out, inhale, press firmly through your hands, straighten your arms, and lengthen your spine forward to create a flat back. Bring your head up so your neck is in line with your spine. Place your hands on your hips, then using your abdominal muscles, bend your knees slightly and raise your torso.

Things to be mindful of: Don't relax in the forward bend. Keep your abdominals pulled in to protect your back. Think of your calves pulling downward and your thighs pulling upward.

Move into . . .

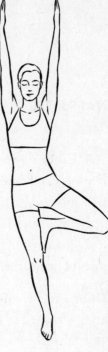

TREE POSE
Vrksasana

1. Stand in mountain pose (*tadasana*) (page 201). Shift your weight onto your left foot, bend your right knee, and with your right hand grab your right ankle. Place the sole of your right foot against your left inner thigh as close to your groin as possible and with toes pointing down. To steady yourself, press the sole of your right foot deeply into your left inner thigh and resist it with your leg.

2. Place your hands on your hips. As you gain balance, raise your arms above your head and, if possible, look up at your hands. Stay in the pose for 5 breaths.

3. Exhale and slide your right foot down your left leg to reach the floor. Repeat on the other side.

Things to be mindful of: Keep your pelvis right under your shoulders and lengthen your tailbone toward the floor. Think about moving your lifted thigh back so it's in the same plane as your torso.

Move into . . .

SUN SALUTATION B
Surya Namaskar B

Come to *tadasana* (page 201). Do 1 *sun salutation B* (page 204). Stay in the pose for 5 breaths.

Move into . . .

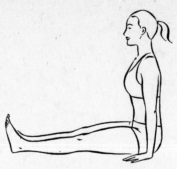

STAFF POSE
Dandasana

1. Come down to the floor and sit with your legs together in front of you, feet flexed. Keep your spine perpendicular to the floor and gaze forward. If this is too challenging, sit on a folded blanket to elevate your pelvis.

2. Place your hands flat on either side of your hips. Stay in this pose for 5 breaths.

Things to be mindful of: As you did in *mountain pose*, imagine a string attached to the top of your head is pulling upward. At the same time, imagine your tailbone lengthening into the floor.

Move into . . .

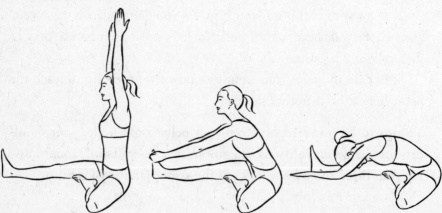

HEAD-TO-KNEE FORWARD BEND A
Janu Sirsasana A

1. Bend your left knee and rest the sole of your left foot against your inner right thigh, placing your heel as high up your thigh as it can comfortably go. Keep your right foot lightly flexed.

2. Inhale, roll your shoulders back, broaden your chest, raise your arms, then lean forward with a straight back to grasp your right foot. If that's too challenging, lay your hands lightly on your shin. Exhale and fold over your right leg, reaching your belly toward your thigh and allowing your arms to fall to either side of your outstretched leg. Stay in the pose for 5 breaths.

3. Inhale to come up and repeat on the other side.

Things to be mindful of: Don't force the stretch. Allow your body to ease farther forward with every exhale.

Move into . . .

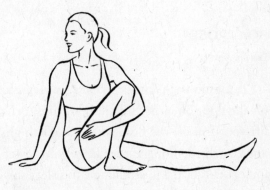

MARICHI'S TWIST C
Marichyasana C

1. Come back into *staff pose* (*dandasana*). Exhale and bend your right leg, placing your heel close to your right sitting bone. Place your right fingertips or palm on the floor behind your right hip and hug your knee with your left arm. If you don't feel much of a stretch, bend your left arm and place your elbow against the outside of your right knee. (You can use the resistance as a lever to help you twist.)

2. Keeping your spine long, inhale, gaze over your right shoulder, and gently rotate your torso to the right. Stay in the pose for 5 breaths.

3. Repeat on the other side.

Things to be mindful of: Keep your abdominal muscles pulled in and see if you can increase the twist slightly on each exhale.

Move into . . .

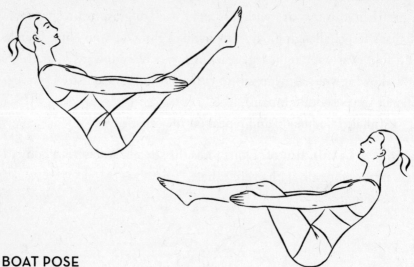

BOAT POSE
Navasana

1. Come back into *staff pose* (*dandasana*). With your hands flat on the floor on either side of your hips, exhale, bend your knees, and lift your feet off the floor so that your thighs are at about a 45-degree angle with the floor. Either keep your lower legs parallel to the floor, knees bent, or try to straighten your legs so your body creates a V. Use your abdominal muscles to keep your legs elevated.

2. Lift your arms alongside your legs at shoulder height and reach through your fingertips. Balance on your sitting bones. Stay in the pose for 5 breaths or as long as possible.

3. Release your arms and legs and come into a cross-legged position with your hands flat on the floor on either side of your hips. Press down with your hands, lifting your body off the floor an inch or two if you're able (if not, just press down on the floor, keeping your legs on the floor).

Do 3 times.

Things to be mindful of: If you feel strain in your lower back while legs are extended, bend your knees.

Move into . . .

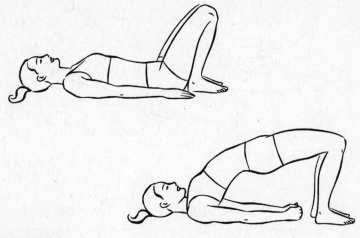

BRIDGE POSE
Setu Bandha Sarvangasana

1. Lie flat on the floor, arms by your side. Bend your knees and place your feet flat on the floor as close to your sitting bones as possible.

2. Exhale, press down on your feet and raise your tailbone off the floor, firming, but not clenching your buttocks, until your thighs are about parallel to the floor. Press upward with your pubic bone.

3. Clasp your hands together on the floor (or just keep your arms parallel to each other if that's more comfortable) below your sitting bones and come up to the tops of your shoulders. Keep your head flat on the floor. Lengthen your arms toward you feet and press down on them to lift the back of your body higher. Stay in the pose for 5 breaths.

4. Exhale and roll your spine down to come back to the floor. Hug your knees into your chest to release your back.

Things to be mindful of: Keep your knees directly above your ankles and think about reaching your shoulder blades down your back so they don't inch up near your ears.

Move into . . .

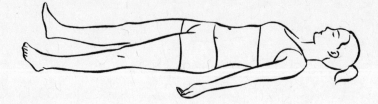

CORPSE POSE
Savasana

1. Work your way to lying flat on the floor. Turn your arms outward and rest them slightly away from your body. Separate your legs about shoulder width apart and let your feet roll outward. Wriggle your back and shoulders until you feel comfortable and grounded on the floor. Close your eyes. Starting with your forehead and moving toward your feet, go through your body and imagine each part releasing. Breathe and relax. Stay in the pose 5 minutes.

2. To come out of the pose, open your eyes, exhale, and roll to your right side. Take a few breaths, then press your hands against the floor and raise your torso, moving into a sitting position.

Namaste!

Resources

······

Slow Money
PO Box 2231
Boulder, CO 80306
info@slowmoney.org
slowmoney.org

Social Venture Network
PO Box 29221
San Francisco, CA 94129
svn.org

1% for the Planet
45 Bridge St
PO Box 650
Waitsfield, VT 05673
info@onepercentfortheplanet.org
onepercentfortheplanet.org

B Corp
155 East Lancaster Avenue
2nd Floor
Wayne, PA 19087
thelab@bcorporation.net
Bcorporation.net

References

......

Agrawal, Rahul, and Fernando Gomez-Pinilla. "'Metabolic Syndrome' in the Brain: Deficiency in Omega-3 Fatty Acid Exacerbates Dysfunctions in Insulin Receptor Signalling and Cognition." *Journal of Physiology* 590 (2012): 2485–99.

Akers, Adam, Jo Barton, Rachel Cossey, Patrick Gainsford, Murray Griffin, and Dominic Micklewright. "Visual Color Perception in Green Exercise: Positive Effects on Mood and Perceived Exertion." *Environmental Science & Technology* 46 (2012): 8661–66.

Albergotti, Reed. "The NFL's Top-Secret Seed; Baltimore Running Back Ray Rice Puts His Faith in Chia Seeds, a Training Tool of the Ancient Aztecs." *Wall Street Journal (Online)*, January 19, 2012.

Albert, Christine M., Kyungwon Oh, William Whang, JoAnn E. Manson, Claudia U. Chae, Meir J. Stampfer, Walter C. Willett, and Frank B. Hu. "Dietary Linolenic Acid Intake and Risk of Sudden Cardiac Death and Coronary Heart Disease." *Circulation* 112 (2005): 3232–38.

Ali, Norlaily Mohd, Swee Keong Yeap, Wan Yong Ho, Boon Kee Beh, Sheau Wei Tan, and Soon Guan Tan. "The Promising Future of Chia, *Salvia hispanica* L." *Journal of Biomedicine and Biotechnology*. Published online November 21, 2012.

Asami, Danny K., Yun-Jeong Hong, Diane M. Barrett, and Alyson E. Mitchell. "Comparison of the Total Phenolic and Ascorbic Acid Content of Freeze-Dried and Air-Dried Marionberry, Strawberry, and Corn Grown Using Conventional, Organic, and Sustainable Agricultural Practices." *Journal of Agricultural and Food Chemistry* 51 no. 5 (2003): 1237–41.

Aspinall, Peter, Panagiotis Mavros, Richard Coyne, and Jenny Roe. "The Urban Brain: Analysing Outdoor Physical Activity with Mobile EEG." *British Journal of Sports Medicine*, March 6, 2013.

Ayerza, Ricardo, Jr., and Wayne Coates. *Chia.* Tucson: University of Arizona Press, 2005.

———. "Effect of Dietary A-Linolenic fatty acid Derived from Chia When Fed as Ground Seed, Whole Seed and Oil on Lipid Content and Fatty Acid Composition of Rat Plasma. *Annals of Nutrition &Metabolism* 51 (2007): 27–34.

Bagga, Dilprit, Karl H. Anders, He-Jing Wang, and John A. Glaspy. "Long-Chain n-3-to-n-6 Polyunsaturated Fatty Acid Ratios in Breast Adipose Tissue From Women With and Without Breast Cancer." *Nutrition and Cancer* 42, no. 2 (2002): 180–85.

Barrett, Bruce, Mary S. Hayney, Daniel Muller, David Rakel, Ann Ward, Chidi N. Obasi, Roger Brown, Zhengjun Zhang, Aleksandra Zgierska, James Gern, Rebecca West, Tola Ewers, Shari Barlow, Michele Gassman, and Christopher L. Coe. "Meditation or Exercise for Preventing Acute Respiratory Infection: A Randomized Controlled Trial." *Annals of Family Medicine* 10, no. 4 (2012): 337–46.

Berkeley Law. "Berkeley Initiative for Mindfulness in Law." July 6, 2013, http://www.law.berkeley.edu/mindfulness.htm.

Borgonovi, Francesca. "Doing Well by Doing Good: The Relationship Between Formal Volunteering and Self-Reported Health and Happiness." *Social Science & Medicine* 66 (2008): 2321–34.

Cahill, Joseph P. 2003. "Ethnobotany of Chia, *Salvia hispanica* L. (Lamiaceae)." *Economic Botany* 57, no. 4 (2003): 604–18.

Calderón-Montaño, J.M., E. Burgos-Morón, C. Perez-Guerrero, and M. López-Lazaro. A Review on the Dietary Flavonoid Kaempferol." *Mini-Reviews in Medicinal Chemistry* 11, no. 4 (2011): 298–344.

Carter, Sherrie Bourg. "Emotions Are Contagious—Choose Your Company Wisely." *Psychology Today,* October 20, 2012. http://www.psychology today.com/blog/high-octane-women/201210/emotionsare-contagious-choose-your-company-wisely.

Cho, Ae-Sim, Seon-Min Jeon, Myung-Joo Kim, Jiyoung Yeo, Kwon-Il Seo, Myung-Sook Choi, and Mi-Kyung Lee. "Chlorogenic Acid Exhibits Anti-Obesity Property and Improves Lipid Metabolism in High-Fat Diet-Induced-Obese Mice." *Food and Chemical Toxicology* 48, no. 3(2010): 937–43.

Cline, Sarah. "Aztecs." In *Encyclopedia of Genocide and Crimes Against Humanity,* ed. Dinah L. Shelton. Vol 1.: 104–107. Macmillan Reference USA, 2005.

Coates, Wayne. *Chia: The Complete Guide to the Ultimate Superfood.* New York: Sterling, 2012.

Condon, Paul, Gaelle Desbordes, Willa B. Miller, and David DeSteno. "Meditation Increases Compassionate Responses to Suffering." *Psychological Science* 24, no. 10 (2013): 2125–27.

Creswell, David J., Michael R. Irwin, Lisa J. Burklund, Matthew D. Lieberman, Jesusa M. G. Arevalo, Jeffrey Ma, Elizabeth Crabb Breen, and Steven W. Cole. "Mindfulness-Based Stress Reduction Training Reduces Loneliness and Pro-Inflammatory Gene Expression in Older Adults: A Small Randomized Controlled Trial." *Brain, Behavior, and Immunity* 26, no. 7 (2012): 1095–1101.

Davis, J. Mark, Catherine J. Carlstedt, Stephen Chen, Martin D. Carmichael, and E. Angela Murphy. "The Dietary Flavonoid Quercetin Increases VO$_2$max and Endurance Capacity." *International Journal of Sport Nutrition and Exercise Metabolism* 20, no. 1 (2010): 58–62.

DeSteno, David. "The Morality of Meditation." *New York Times,* July 5, 2013. http://www.nytimes.com/2013/07/07/opinion/sunday/the-moralityof-meditation.html?_r=0.

Douglas, Steve M., Laura C. Ortinau, Heather A. Hoertel, and Heather J. Leidy. "Low, Moderate, or High Protein Yogurt Snacks on Appetite Control and Subsequent Eating in Healthy Women." *Appetite* 60, no. 1 (2013): 117–22.

Edenfield, Teresa M., and Sy Atezaz Saeed. "An Update on Mindfulness Meditation as a Self-Help Treatment for Anxiety and Depression." *Psychology Research and Behavior Management* 5 (2012): 131–41.

Ekkekakis, Panteleimon, Gaynor Parfitt, and Steven J. Petruzzello. "The Pleasure and Displeasure People Feel When They Exercise at Different Intensities: Decennial Update and Progress Towards a Tripartite Rationale for Exercise Intensity Prescription." *Sports Medicine* 41, no. 8 (2011): 641–71.

Environmental Working Group. "Frequently Asked Questions About Produce and Pesticides." Accessed July 10, 2013. http://www.ewg.org/foodnews/faq.php#note_1.

Flower, Kori B., Jane A. Hoppin, Charles F. Lynch, Aaron Blair, Charles Knott, David L. Shore, and Dale P. Sandler. "Cancer Risk and Parental Pesticide Application in Children of Agricultural Health Study Participants." *Environmental Health Perspectives* 112, no. 5 (2004): 631–35.

Goodland, Robert and Jeff Anhang. "Livestock and Climate Change: What

If the Key Actors in Climate Change Are . . . Cows, Pigs, and Chickens?" *World Watch,* November/December 2009. http://www.world watch.org/files/pdf/Livestock%20and%20Climate%20Change.pdf.

Guiney, Hayley and Liana Machado. "Benefits of Regular Aerobic Exercise for Executive Functioning in Healthy Populations." *Psychonomic Bulletin & Review* 20, no. 1(2013): 73–86.

Harvard School of Public Health. "Fiber: Start Roughing It!" http://www .hsph.harvard.edu/nutritionsource/fiber-full-story/.

Ho, H., A. S. Lee, E. Jovanovski, A. L. Jenkins, R. DeSouza, and V. Vuksan. "Effect of Whole and Ground Salba Seeds (*Salvia Hispanic* L.) on Postprandial Glycemia in Healthy Volunteers: a Randomized Controlled, Dose-Response Trial." *European Journal of Clinical Nutrition* 67 (2013): 786–88.

Holt-Lunstad, Julianne, Timothy B. Smith, and J. Bradley Layton. "Social Relationships and Mortality Risk: A Meta-analytic Review." *PLoS Med* 7, no. 7 (2010): e1000316.

Hughes, J. D. "The European Biotic Invasion of Aztec Mexico." *Capitalism, Nature, Socialism* 11, no. 1 (2000): 105.

Illian, Travis G., Jason C. Casey, and Phillip A. Bishop. "Omega 3 Chia Seed Loading as a Means Of Carbohydrate Loading." *Journal of Strength and Conditioning Research* 25, no. 1 (2011): 61–65.

Jaremka, Lisa M., Christopher P. Fagundes, Juan Peng, Jeanette M. Bennett, Ronald Glaser, William B. Malarkey, and Janice K. Kiecolt-Glaser. "Loneliness Promotes Inflammation During Acute Stress." *Psychological Science* 24, no. 7 (2013): 1089–97.

Jeong, Se Kyoo, Hyun Jung Park, Byeong Deog Park, and Il-Hwan Kim. "Effectiveness of Topical Chia Seed Oil on Pruritus of End-stage Renal Disease (ESRD) Patients and Healthy Volunteers." *Annals of Dermatology* 22, no. 2 (2010): 13–148.

Jin, Fuxia, David C. Nieman, Wei Sha, Guoxiang Xie, Yunping Qiu, and Wei Jia. "Supplementation of Milled Chia Seeds Increases Plasma ALA and EPA in Postmenopausal Women." *Plant Foods for Human Nutrition* 67 (2012): 105–10.

Kelly, Caitlin. "O.K., Google, Take a Deep Breath." *New York Times,* April 28, 2012. http://www.nytimes.com/2012/04/29/technology/google-course -asks-employees-to-take-a-deep-breath.html?pagewanted=all&_r=0.

Kiecolt-Glaser, Janice K., Martha A. Belury, Rebecca Andridge, William B. Malarkey, Beom Seuk Hwang, and Ronald Glaser. "Omega-3 Supplementation Lowers Inflammation in Healthy Middle-Aged and Older Adults: A Randomized Controlled Trial." *Brain, Behavior and Immunity* 26, no. 6 (2012): 988–95.

Koh, Eunmi, Suthawan Charoenprasert, and Alyson E. Mitchell. "Effect of Organic and Conventional Cropping Systems on Ascorbic Acid, Vitamin C, Flavonoids, Nitrate, and Oxalate in 27 Varieties of Spinach (*Spinacia oleracea* L.)." *Journal of Agricultural and Food Chemistry* 60, no. 12 (2012): 3144–50.

Kraft, Tara L., and Sarah D. Pressman. "Grin and Bear It: The Influence of Manipulated Facial Expression on the Stress Response." *Psychological Science* 23, no. 11 (2012): 1372–78.

Label GMOs. "What Are We Eating?" http://www.labelgmos.org/the_science_genetically_modified_foods_gmo.

Lavretsky, H., E. S. Epel, P. Siddarth, N. Nazarian, N. St. Cyr, D. S. Khalsa, J. Lin, E. Blackburn, and M. R. Irwin. "A Pilot Study of Yogic Meditation for Family Dementia Caregivers with Depressive Symptoms: Effects on Mental Health, Cognition, and Telomerase Activity." *International Journal of Geriatric Psychiatry* 28, no. 1 (2013): 57–65.

Lippert, Marissa. "Organic or Not? Is Organic Produce Healthier Than Conventional?" *Eating Well.* http://www.eatingwell.com/food_news_origins/green_sustainable/organicor_nois_organic_produce_healthier_than_conventional.

Luders, Eileen, Kristi Clark, Katherine L. Narr, and Arthur W. Toga. "Enhanced Brain Connectivity in Long-term Meditation Practitioners." *Neuroimage* 57, no. 4 (2011): 1308–16.

Mangat, Iqwall. "Do Vegetarians Have to Eat Fish for Optimal Cardiovascular Protection?" *American Journal of Clinical Nutrition* 89, no. 5 (2009): 15975–16015.

McDougall, Christopher. *Born to Run: A Hidden Tribe, Superathletes, and the Greatest Race the World Has Never Seen.* New York: Vintage, 2009.

Melnick, Meredith. "Meditation Health Benefits: What the Practice Does to Your Body." *Huffington Post,* April 2, 2013. http://www.huffingtonpost.com/2013/04/30/meditation-health benefits_n_3178731.html.

Novaes, Rômulo D, Reggiani V. Gonçalves, Maria do Carmo G. Peluzio, Antônio J. Natali, and Izabel R. S. C. Maldonado. "3,4-Dihydroxycinnamic Acid Attentuates the Fatigue and Improves Exercise Tolerance in Rats." *Bioscience, Biotechnology, Biochemistry* 76, no. 5 (2012): 1025–27.

Orchard, Tonya S., Steven Wing, Bo Lu, Martha A. Belury, Karen Johnson,

Jean Wactawski-Wende, and Rebecca D. Jackson. "The Association of Red Blood Cell n-3 and n-6 Fatty Acids with Bone Mineral Density and Hip Fracture Risk in the Women's Health Initiative." *Journal of Bone and Mineral Research* 28, no. 3 (2013): 505–15.

Organic Trade Association. "Antibiotics in Agriculture." 2013. http://www .ota.com/organic/benefits/antibiotics.html.

———. "Eight in Ten U.S. Parents Report They Purchase Organic Products," July, 2008. http://www.organicnewsroom.com/2013/04/eight_ in_ten_us_parents_report.html.

———. "Impacts of Toxic and Persistent Chemicals Due to Non Organic Operations," October 2008. http://www.ota.com/organic/health/ environment/consumers/exposure.html?printable=1.

———. "Organic Agriculture and Production," April 1, 2013. http://www .ota.com/definition/quickoverview.html.

Palmer, Sharon. "Is There a Link Between Nutrition and Autoimmune Disease?" *Today's Dietitian* 13, no. 11 (2011): 36.

Perrone, Matthew. "Does Giving Antibiotics to Animals Hurt Humans?" April 20, 2012. http://usatoday30.usatoday.com/news/health/story/ 2012-04-20/antibioticsanimals-human-meat/54434860/1.

Post, Stephen G. "Altruism, Happiness, and Health: It's Good to Be Good." *International Journal of Behavioral Medicine* 12, no. 2 (2005): 66–77.

Rauzi, Robin. "Tapping Into the Power of Mindfulness." *Los Angeles Times,* February 23, 2013. http://articles.latimes.com/2013/feb/23/business/la- fi-meditation management 20130224.

Robinson, Jo. *Eating on the Wild Side.* New York: Little, Brown and Company, 2013.

Rolls, Barbara, and Robert A. Barnett. *The Volumetrics Weight-Control Plan.* New York: Harper Collins, 2000.

Sandoval-Oliveros, Maria R., and Octavio Paredes-López. "Isolation and Characterization of Proteins from Chia Seeds (*Salvia hispanica* L.)." *Journal of Agriculture and Food Chemistry* 61, no. 1 (2013): 193–201.

Sax, David. "Chia Seeds, Wall Street's Stimulant of Choice." *Bloomberg Business Week,* May 24, 2012. http://www.businessweek.com/ articles/2012-05-24/chia-seeds-wall-streets-stimulant-of-choice.

Schley, Patricia D., Humberto J. Jijon, Lindsay E. Robinson, and Catherine J. Field. "Mechanisms of Omega-3 Fatty Acid-Induced Growth Inhibition in MDA-MB-231 Human Breast Cancer Cells." *Breast Cancer Research and Treatment* 92, no. 2 (2005): 187–95.

Simopoulous, Artemis P. "Omega-3 Fatty Acids in Inflammation and Auto-immune Diseases." *Journal of the American College of Nutrition* 21, no. 6 (2002): 495–505.

Singh, Ram B., Gal Dubnov, Mohammad A. Niaz, Saraswati Ghosh, Reema Singh, Shanti S Rastogi, Orly Manor, Daniel Pella, and Elliot M. Berry. "Effect of an Indo-Mediterranean Diet on Progression of Coronary Artery Disease in High Risk Patients (Indo-Mediterranean Diet Heart Study): A Randomised Single Blind Trial." *Lancet* 360, no. 9344 (2002): 1455–61.

Smith-Spangler, Crystal, Margaret L. Brandeau, Grace E. Hunter, J. Clay Bavinger, Maren Pearson, Paul J. Eschbach, Vandana Sundaram, Hau Liu, Patricia Schirmer, Christopher Stave, Ingram Olkin, and Dena M. Bravata. "Are Organic Foods Safer or Healthier than Conventional Alternatives?: A Systematic Review." *Annals of Internal Medicine* 157, no. 5 (2012): 348–66.

SoundaraPandian, Shenbaga; Panteleimon Ekkekakis; and Amy S. Welch. "Exercise as an Affective Experience: Does Adding a Positive End Impact Future Exercise Choice?" *Medicine & Science in Sports & Exercise* 42, no. 5 (2010): 102–103.

Steinberg, Hannah, Elizabeth A. Sykes, Tim Moss, Susan Lowery, Nick LeBoutillier, and Alison Dewey. 1997. "Exercise Enhances Creativity Independently of Mood." *British Journal of Sports Medicine* 31, no. 3 (1997): 240–45.

Timbrook, Jan. "Chia and the Chumas: A Reconsideration for Sage Seeds in Southern California." *Journal of California and Great Basin Anthropology* 8, no. 1 (1986): 50–64.

Toohey, A. M., G. R. McCormack, P. K. Doyle-Baker, C. L. Adams, and M. J. Rock. "Dog-Walking and Sense of Community in Neighborhoods: Implications for Promoting Regular Physical Activity in Adults 50 Years and Older." *Health & Place* 22 (2013): 75–81.

United States Department of Agriculture Natural Resources Conservation Service. "Plant Guide: Chia: *Salvia columbariae* Benth," 2003. http://plants.usda.gov/plantguide/doc/cs_saco6.docx.

Voss, Michelle W., Ruchika S. Prakash, Kirk I. Erickson, Chandramallika Basak, Laura Chaddock, Jennifer S. Kim, Heloisa Alves, Susie Heo, Amanda N. Szabo, Siobhan M. White, Thomas R. Wójcikcki, Emily L. Mailey, Neha Gothe, Erin A. Olson, Edward McAuley, and Arthur F. Kramer. "Plasticity of Brain Networks in a Randomized Intervention

Trial of Exercise Training in Older Adults." *Frontiers in Aging Neuroscience* 2 (2010): 32.

Vuksan, Vladimir, Dana Whitham, John L. Sievenpiper, Alexandra L. Jenkins, Alexander L. Rogovik, Richard Pl Bazinet, Edward Vidgen, and Amir Hanna. "Supplementation of Conventional Therapy with the Novel Grain Salba (*Salvia hispanica* L.) Improves Major Emerging Cardiovascular Risk Factors in Type 2 Diabetes." *Diabetes Care* (2007): 2804–10.

Walton, G. M., G. L. Cohen, D. Cwir, and S. J. Spence. "Mere Belonging: The Power of Social Connections." *Journal of Personality and Social Psychology* 102, no. 3 (2012): 513–32.

Welch, Ailsa, Subodha Shakya-Shrestha, Marleen A. H. Lentjes, Nicholas J. Wareham, and Kay-Tee Khaw. "Dietary Intake and Status of N-3 Polyunsaturated Fatty Acids in a Population of Fish-Eating and Non-Fish-Eating Meat-Eaters, Vegetarians, and Vegans and the Precursor-Product Ratio of a-Linolenic Acid to Long-Cahin N-3 Polyunsaturated Fatty Acids: Results from the EPIC-Norfolk Cohort." *American Journal of Clinical Nutrition* 92, no. 5 (2010): 1040–51.

Westerterp-Plantenga, Sofie G. Lemmens, and Klaas R. Westerterp. "Dietary Protein–Its Role in Satiety, Energetics, Weight Loss and Health." *British Journal of Nutrition* 108 (2012): S105–S112.

Willett, Walter C. *Eat, Drink, and Be Healthy: The Harvard Medical School Guide to Healthy Eating.* New York: Fireside, 2001.

Wright, S. A., F. M. O'Prey, M. T. McHenry, W. J. Leahey, A. B. Devine, E. M. Duffy, D. G. Johnston, M.B. Finch, A. L. Bell, and G. E. McVeigh. "A Randomized Interventional Trial of Omega-3 Polyunsaturated Fatty Acids on Endothelial Function and Disease Activity in Systemic Lupus Erythematosus." *Annals of the Rheumatic Diseases* 67, no. 6 (2008): 841–48.

Index

Hungry for More?

• • • • • •

Janie Hoffman presents a colorful recipe collection that takes cooking with chia to the next level, with hearty and healthy breakfast, lunch, dinner, snacks, and sweets.

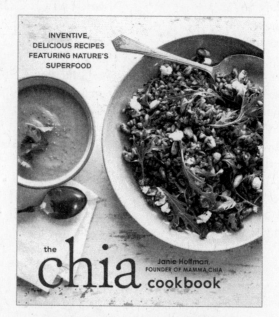

THE CHIA COOKBOOK
Inventive, Delicious Recipes
Featuring Nature's Superfood

WWW.TENSPEED.COM

Available on September 30, 2014, from Ten Speed Press,
wherever books are sold